THE VITAMIN CURE

for Allergies

DAMIEN DOWNING, M.D.

Basic
Health
PUBLICATIONS, INC.

The information contained in this book is based upon the research and personal and professional experiences of the authors. It is not intended as a substitute for consulting with your physician or other healthcare provider. Any attempt to diagnose and treat an illness should be done under the direction of a healthcare professional.

The publisher does not advocate the use of any particular healthcare protocol but believes the information in this book should be available to the public. The publisher and authors are not responsible for any adverse effects or consequences resulting from the use of the suggestions, preparations, or procedures discussed in this book. Should the reader have any questions concerning the appropriateness of any procedures or preparation mentioned, the authors and the publisher strongly suggest consulting a professional healthcare advisor.

Basic Health Publications, Inc.
28812 Top of the World Drive
Laguna Beach, CA 92651
949-715-7327 • www.basichealthpub.com

Library of Congress Cataloging-in-Publication Data
Downing, Damien.
    The vitamin cure for allergies / Damien Downing.
        p. cm.
    Includes bibliographical references and index.
    ISBN 978-1-59120-271-4
    1. Allergy—Popular works. 2. Vitamin therapy—Popular works.
I. Title.
    RC585.D69   2010
    615'.328—dc22
                                                    2010018684

Editor: John Anderson
Typesetting/Book design: Gary A. Rosenberg
Cover design: Mike Stromberg

Printed in the United States of America

10   9   8   7   6   5   4   3   2   1

CONTENTS

INTRODUCTION

Allergies are no fun. I know this because I spent my high school years spaced out on antihistamines every summer, otherwise I wouldn't have been able to see the exam papers because of sneezing and watering eyes. And that was a long time ago; believe me, allergies have gotten a lot worse since then (but I'm much better, thank you for asking). Experts now admit we're in an allergy epidemic.

Throughout the developed world, the number of people with allergies has been rising for fifty years—and rising steeply for the last twenty years. Everybody is at risk. There's been a massive increase in children with a dangerous peanut allergy; in fact, kids are the worst hit with all allergies. Every year, the U.S. Centers for Disease Control and Prevention, in Atlanta, carries out a National Health Interview Survey. Two years ago, they focused on allergies and found that between 1999 and 2005, the number of those under eighteen years old being admitted to the hospital with allergies more than trebled in just six years.[1]

Our medical system can't cope—many allergy cases are misdiagnosed and people often don't find relief even when they are treated. Or if they are helped by drugs, it's often at too high a price in side effects.

The good news is that there is so much you can do for yourself to make allergies better, and this book will help you.

1

THE MISERY OF ALLERGIES

You're probably already familiar with the misery that allergies can cause. Symptoms can include sneezing, itching, bloating, and headaches. Severe allergic reactions can even cause anaphylactic shock, which, if left untreated, could lead to death.

Allergies can be caused by a wide variety of things. The most common categories are:

- Inhalants—pollen, animal dander, molds, etc.

- Foods—wheat and milk are the most common examples.

- Chemicals—solvents, gasoline, smoke, perfumes, etc.

WHAT CAN BE DONE?

Fortunately, there are a number of things you can do to help prevent and relieve your allergies.

Avoid

Once you have figured out what sets you off, stay away from it. Obvious, but not always simple. How do you avoid pollen in high summer? Or mold in a damp house? How do you stay off bread and all wheat products when you're trying to feed a hungry family? We'll answer these questions.

You also want to remove anything to which you react, not only from your environment but from your body too. This is most important with the chemicals, where you may need special detoxification methods to get them out. Foods generally take around forty-eight hours to pass through the gut, and for all that time you are potentially exposed to them and may react. We'll discuss diets, detoxing, and supplements and herbs that can help.

Protect

You can use nutrition to damp down the symptoms of allergies when they happen, and also to prevent them from happening in the first place. A number of nutrients have proven effective in treating allergies, including vitamins C and D, essential fatty acids, and magnesium. I'll tell you when it's safe to use nutrition, and when it's likely to be effective.

Desensitize

When all else fails, or doesn't work well enough, you can consider desensitization techniques. Like a vaccination, desensitization involves giving a small dose of something to which you are allergic in order to reduce your immune system's reaction. There are a number of desensitization options, including homeopathic formulas, neutralization, and enzyme-potentiated desensitization (EPD). These aren't always successful (any more than vaccination is), but there's probably an excellent chance that one of these techniques will work for you.

YOU CAN FIND RELIEF FROM ALLERGIES

I'm a doctor, qualified in 1972, and living and working in London. I left the British National Health Service in 1980 to get back my clinical freedom—the right to treat patients in the way the patient and I agreed was best, not according to some official "guideline." I'm now in an integrated medicine team with other doctors, including a naturopath, an osteopath, and a Chinese medicine specialist. I'm also the president of the British Society for Ecological Medicine, and I spend a great deal of time researching and writing about the environment and our health.

I have seen many patients with allergies and sensitivities, and I've treated them with many of the methods that are explained in this book. I've seen these treatments work and provide profound relief to patients in my practice. I am confident that by reading this book and incorporating these methods into your own life, you too will find relief from your allergies.

CHAPTER 1

WHAT IS AN ALLERGY?

A textbook definition of allergy has been argued about among doctors and scientists for over a hundred years now. Just during the time that I've been a doctor, we have seen the idea of food allergies come out of nowhere to be accepted, although the "old guard" of doctors still like to restrict the term allergy to symptoms like asthma and eczema, and they refer to "food intolerances" rather than food allergies. If you suffer from allergies, you don't give a hoot what they call it. In this book, I'm going to cover allergies, intolerances, sensitivities, and anything else you like to call them, so the exact medical definitions don't work. The dictionary definition of allergy is a damaging immune response by the body to a substance, especially pollen, fur, food, or dust, to which it has become hypersensitive. In other words, an allergy is any encounter with something from the environment that gives you symptoms.

How do you know it's an allergy? Common allergy symptoms may include sneezing, wheezing, itching, bloating, cramps, lack of energy, sleepiness, irritability, trouble concentrating, and headaches. But each of these can be caused by other things than allergies, so an allergy should be suspected when exposure to something in particular gives you the symptoms. For example, you walk through a park and start to sneeze; or you eat eggs or another food and you start to bloat; or you get in a taxi with one of those air fresheners and you get a sore throat or a headache.

TYPES OF ALLERGIES

There are three common categories of things to which you can be allergic: inhalants, foods, and chemicals.

Inhalants

Pollens, animal fur, molds, and dust mites are the main inhalants. They are carried from plants and animals through the air, and you breathe them in. The "portal of entry" is the nose and throat (and eyes), and this is where the symptoms happen, mostly. These are the "classic" allergies that conventional medicine has recognized for a long time, and it has a reasonable understanding of the mechanisms involved. These types of allergies barely existed back before humans developed industry and its subsequent pollution, and they still happen more in urban areas than in the country. But only now are we starting to understand why.

Foods

There probably isn't a single food that has never caused an allergic reaction, but the ones that cause the most allergies are the ones that appear most in our diet, and particularly the ones that are in prepared foods, often without you knowing about it. Wheat and milk products are at the top of the list, along with food colorings. Twenty-five years ago, most doctors thought the idea that people might have allergies to foods was ridiculous, but now they have to admit it is real. Allergists still like to call most reactions to foods "intolerances" to distinguish them from the classic allergies, which is fair enough for a scientist looking at mechanisms, but does nothing for the sufferer. It should never be used to suggest that intolerances are less serious.

Chemicals

Solvents, perfumes, gasoline and exhaust fumes, tobacco smoke, and cleaning fluids are the primary culprits. Strictly speaking,

ALLERGIES, INTOLERANCES, OR SENSITIVITIES?

A lot of hot air has been expended on debating the right word to use for reactions to foods in particular. Some conventional allergists have argued that the term *allergy* should only be used to refer to classic allergies (atopy, immediate hypersensitivity). The diseases in this group include asthma, eczema, hay fever, urticaria (hives), angioedema, reactions to insect bites or stings, and certain immediate reactions to foods. Everything else is excluded. Others have argued that when the word *allergy* was first used a century ago, by a Vienna pediatrician named von Pirquet, it covered every kind of adverse reaction. The word, from the Greek words *allos* and *ergos* ("different work"), simply means an altered response.

I have to admit to fudging this one. I generally talk about food intolerances when I'm talking to other doctors, because I know it's important to them, but I talk about food allergies when discussing them with patients/sufferers, because they couldn't care less about such petty arguments, they just want to feel well. In this book, I use the two terms for reactions to foods interchangeably.

we're talking about chemical fumes, things that you breathe in and smell—and if you react to it, you may well be much more sensitive to the smell. We now know that some of us have genes that are less good at making the important liver enzymes that detoxify our system. This can make you much more likely to develop chemical sensitivities.[1] Of course, if you can't get rid of a chemical, it may stay in your system for a long time, making you ill.

Other Categories

Drug allergies—Drug allergies can be dangerous because they can cause severe reactions such as anaphylaxis and Stevens-Johnson

ELECTROSENSITIVITY

Electrosensitivity (ES) and electrohypersensitivity (EHS) are some of the names used to describe a recent phenomenon. As a practitioner, I'm actually quite cautious—I'm happy to let other people be the guinea pigs before I use something on my patients. It has therefore taken me thirty years of practicing medicine to get to the point where I can write this book. I first became persuaded that food intolerances were real back in the early 1980s (taught by my patients, as usual). It has taken the medical profession years to catch up, and even now I come across the occasional doctor who "doesn't believe" in them. It took about another decade to convince me that chemical sensitivities were real; most of medicine is deep in denial about them right now. Electrosensitivity is way behind that, and it is only in the last few years that I've come to accept it, and it will be a long time before scientists and doctors in general do.

It's only become a problem since everybody started acquiring a mobile phone and a WiFi, simply because there are more electromagnetic fields (EMFs). The inverse square law states that if you double the distance from a transmitter (source of the waves) to yourself, you reduce the energy in the waves (the signal power) by four; treble the distance and you reduce it by nine. So where's the nearest TV broadcast tower to where you are right now? Tens of miles, probably, and twenty-five years ago that was all the EMFs around us. Now, there will be a phone antenna no more than a couple of miles away, and possibly right over your head, and a WiFi base station in the next room. In fact, when I turn on the WiFi detector in my office, I get about thirty different networks I could sign on to.

Most of the people I see who have a problem with EMFs turn out to have a phone antenna just down the block, or a cordless phone, or another nearby source of strong EMFs. If it is a WiFi, they have usually figured it out already and powered it down.

I grant that this is not an allergy in the strictest sense, but it is certainly an altered response to an outside factor. The reason this book doesn't address it is that there is not a lot we can do about it. But that is changing—researchers are identifying what goes on in the body and are developing ways of tackling it.

Syndrome, and they can come on rapidly without warning. We won't discuss them much in this book, simply because they don't usually give you a chance to use vitamins or more natural methods to treat them, and you may have no choice but to use life-saving medicines. They don't usually become chronic because as soon as you figure it out, you never take the medicine again. I do advise wearing a MedicAlert or similar bracelet or card, in case you find yourself in the emergency department and in no state to give them a history.

Organisms—Problems with *Candida* and other yeasts are quite well-known now, but only some of them are allergic. *Candida* is a normal member of the gut flora, the trillions of organisms of dozens of species that live in your large bowel, and they don't cause allergies in most of us. Taking too many antibiotics can disrupt the balance in your intestinal tract and allow *Candida* to flourish; that alone can make you unwell. Sometimes, you may develop an allergy to it as well.

INHALANT ALLERGIES

All types of allergies tend to show first at the "portal of entry," the place that the allergen gets into your body and first activates the immune system. Inhalant allergy symptoms are usually and mainly in the respiratory tract (the nose, throat, and sometimes right down into the lungs).

Symptoms

The main symptoms of inhalant allergies include the following (you don't need them all for a diagnosis—just one will do).

Rhinitis—Inflammation and swelling of the inside of the nose, which can block it and make breathing difficult. A doctor looking into your nose with a light can usually see that the lining is red and swollen.

Rhinorrhea—Production of excessive amounts of mucus (intended to expel the pollen or other allergen), which can flow out through the nostrils and/or back and down the throat, sometimes called "post-nasal drip."

Sneezing—Rapid, explosive exhalations through the nose, also meant to expel allergens, viruses, or other irritants. A sneeze is a reflex (you can't decide not to do it) in which the top of the throat opens up, and at the same time the back of the tongue rises to close off the mouth, so that most of the air expelled has to go through the nose, where it helps to expel the mucus you are producing.

Other symptoms include:

Coughing—Like sneezing, coughing is designed to expel irritants such as allergens, but in this case from further down in the throat and the lungs.

Wheezing—Difficult, audible breathing out. This happens when the tissue of the lungs becomes swollen; it can't expand outward because of the rib cage, so it expands inward, making the bronchioles (the small tubes through which the air flows) narrower. It is the main symptom of asthma, an allergy in the lungs; it also happens sometimes when hay fever or rhinitis is at its most severe.

Conjunctivitis—Inflammation of the lining of the eyes. It feels itchy or prickly, and sometimes sore, and the inside of the eyelids becomes redder and slightly swollen.

Headache—This happens both because the sinuses (cavities in the bones of the face, above and below the eyes) get inflamed and as part of a more general inflammation process.

Malaise—The medical term for feeling ill. It, too, happens when there is inflammation; the body produces messenger molecules called cytokines that activate the immune system, but which also make you feel achy, lethargic, drowsy, and generally lousy.

Causes

Often, the pattern of symptoms in an allergy will tell you what the cause, the allergen, is. This is particularly true with inhalant allergies. Let's look at the common allergens and the symptom patterns they generate.

Pollens

Grass pollen—The most common inhalant allergy in northern Europe is to grass pollen. This allergy happens in high summer (early June through August) in most of the Northern hemisphere, though later and for a shorter time the further north you go. When I was a junior doctor in York in northern England, every summer we would get asthmatics rushed in by ambulance immediately after the local council sent the mowers round to cut the grass, sending loads of pollen into the air.

Ragweed pollen—This is a big allergy in North America, less so in Europe. Ragweed is everywhere in the United States and impossible to eradicate completely. Its pollen is very light and can be carried for hundreds of miles on the wind. The pollen season can run from July through November, with a peak in September.

Tree pollen—In North America, the weather is what's described as "continental," meaning that it's more extreme than in places like Britain, where the sea keeps the winters mild and the summers cool. That's why in New York it seems to be either snowing or sweltering. It also means that Spring happens fast, so most tree pollens arrive no more than a few weeks before the grass pollens. In Britain, it's different—if you get hay fever earlier in the year, in March and April, it'll be due to tree pollen. There are some exceptions to the American rule; for instance there are species of cedar, particularly in the southern Rockies, that pollinate in January to February.

House Dust Mites

House dust mites are invisibly small, eight-legged insects, less than half a millimeter in length, which is just as well because they are ugly little beasts. They live in mattresses, furniture, carpets, and other hidden places, feeding on rotting organic matter, including our skin debris. They like warmth and dampness, which is why going to sleep and breathing warm air into your pillow brings them out to party. This is the only time you're likely to be in close contact with them, so an allergy to dust mites typically happens in the night and is at its worst when you wake up. That's a give-away for the cause of rhinitis. You really don't need to know this, but dust mite feces are produced covered in a membrane or capsule, and it is this, not the animal itself, that causes the allergy in most cases.

Molds

There are thousands of species of mold thriving out there, living on, and by, rotting organic matter. They all produce spores (sporulate), like seeds, that are carried on the air, which is usually how they cause allergies. Of course, some molds are useful, such as the ones that produce the blue color in blue cheese, not to mention the ones that gave us penicillin. But some of them, known as "toxic molds," also produce mycotoxins, molecules that can damage nerves and even kill. This happens when a large growth of toxic mold happens in an indoor, confined space. Because they need a damp and fairly warm environment to sporulate, we tend to think of molds as a problem in the Fall only. While this is true of many molds, it's not true of others. There are molds that grow on grains and are a problem at harvest time; there are ones that use the splash of raindrops to launch them into the air and so are a problem mainly in thunderstorms. There are molds that grow on paper, on paint, on plaster, and on bare wood, so nowhere in a house is guaranteed safe from molds.

Then, there's the garden as a source for molds . . .

Other Factors

It has long been known that inhalant hay fever is more common, and often more severe, in cities than in the countryside, and the reasons are now becoming clear. Pollen grains are very small, around 30 microns (30 thousandths of a millimeter), and can be carried long distances on the wind. But urban and other human-made pollution, from vehicle exhaust or wherever, is even smaller, mostly under 10 microns (known as PM10s, for particulate mat-

THE IMPORTANCE OF MUCOUS MEMBRANES

All the "inside outsides" of your body are mucous membranes, like skin but different. The entire lining of your gut or digestive tract, from lips (which are halfway between skin and mucous membrane) through to anus; the respiratory tract from the nose down into the lungs; the inside of your eyelids; the inside of the vagina and the uterus; the urethra—all of these are mucous membranes. It is moist because of the mucus it produces; it has been estimated that an adult produces about a liter (about a quart) of mucus every day (I have no idea how they calculate that). Mucus has a number of functions: it protects the membrane, forming a slippery film over it; it lubricates (ever noticed how hard it is to swallow with a dry throat?); and it contains enzymes and antibodies that protect against infection.

ter less than 10 microns) and much of it is under 2.5 microns (PM2.5s). When pollen grains are being carried through urban air, they tend to get a load of these smaller pollution particles attached to them. When a "dirty" pollen grain lands in your nose, these particles are even more of an irritant to your mucous membranes than the ordinary pollen and can make hay fever worse. What's more, unlike the pollen, they are small enough to be carried down into the lungs, where they may set off asthma. So it's no surprise to find that increasing levels of pollution, both the particulate matter and sulfur dioxide (SO_2), make hay fever and asthma more common.

Your genetic make-up also plays a part in these allergies. When scientists looked at hay fever sufferers, they found that mixing pollen with exhaust fumes or tobacco smoke increased the amount of IgE antibody they produced by a factor of five. But if the hay fever sufferer had a particular form of one specific gene (known as a polymorphism), this meant they were less effective at getting rid of pollutants and toxins, and the pollution increased their IgE production by fifteen times. So if you're not so good at excreting it, pollution will make your allergy a lot worse.

FOOD ALLERGIES AND INTOLERANCES

In the case of food allergies, the portal of entry is the digestive system, so this is often where the main symptoms occur. As with inhalant allergies, you can get more general, whole-body symptoms as well, but the emphasis is shifted even more this way in food reactions, so general symptoms are more common. Because the digestion and absorption of food into the system only really starts when it reaches the intestine, this is when the symptoms typically begin, maybe 45 to 60 minutes after you start eating. But not always—there is a thankfully uncommon form of reaction called "oral allergy syndrome" in which symptoms start immediately when the allergen touches the lips and can involve dangerous swelling of the mouth and throat. Even smelling the food may cause itching. We'll deal with this potentially serious reaction in Chapter 2: Allergies That Kill.

Symptoms

With the core symptoms of food allergies, you don't need them all for a diagnosis, though having more than two is more definitive. Most of these symptoms are bowel-related, because this is where foods come into the body. You may also note that most of them can have other, nonallergic causes—what *can't* cause fatigue, for instance? Altered bowel habits could be due to stress, infection, even a tumor. And, of course, it is entirely possible to have more than one thing going on: to have an inflamed gut due to an infection or injury, for instance, which allows a food intolerance to develop and inflames the gut even more, and so on. This means that even a strong suspicion of a food intolerance does not abolish the need to rule out other, potentially serious explanations for the symptoms, for which you will need the help of a doctor. This is also why I say you need more than two symptoms to suspect food intolerances.

Bloating—Swelling of the abdomen, usually after food is eaten. This is due to gas (wind) in the bowel. It's not just the most important symptom of food intolerance, it also has consequences. When the bowel is stretched by having gas in it, the pressure can flatten out the tiny finger-like projections of the bowel wall known as villi. Remember when they told you in biology class that if you stretched out the small intestine, it would have the surface area of a tennis court? That's due to all the villi, and you need that surface area to absorb all the nutrients you get from food. When it is flattened, the surface area can reduce by 60 percent, which will impair the complex process of absorbing nutrients.

Wind—Belching or breaking wind, which naturally goes with bloating, and may or may not alleviate it.

Altered bowel habits—Either loose and/or more frequent bowel motions, which when bad we call diarrhea, while harder, less frequent bowel motions are called constipation. Sometimes, symptoms will involve alternating between the two. (See also the inset on Irritable Bowel Syndrome.)

IRRITABLE BOWEL SYNDROME

Irritable bowel syndrome (IBS) or spastic colon is a strange diagnosis. Note, firstly, that it is called a syndrome, not a disease; a syndrome is a cluster of symptoms that tend to go together (the word literally means "run together"). It says nothing about why you get the symptoms, and it means that doctors don't know why. In fact, IBS is a "diagnosis of exclusion": when you've ruled out all the known causes of the symptoms (abdominal pain or discomfort and either diarrhea or constipation), everything left is considered IBS. But these symptoms are very close to those of food intolerance. And if you treat IBS as a food intolerance, it often clears up. I wonder why that is?

Pain or discomfort—Along with the abdominal discomfort that goes with bloating, you can also get quite unpleasant abdominal cramps and spasms with a food reaction; this is true whether you have constipation or diarrhea.

Fatigue, drowsiness—It is true, as I said above, that fatigue can be caused by almost any illness. There's a reason for this: cytokines. These messenger molecules are used by the body to activate the immune system, and they cause you to feel unwell, tired, and sleepy.

Brain symptoms—Fuzzy head (some people call it "the fogs"), impaired concentration and memory, headache, and even difficulty focusing your eyes are all signs of a reaction going on in the brain and nervous system, a target organ for the allergy.

Altered pulse—I mention this because it has been used as a self-administered test for an allergic reaction (Coca's test). It's not a very reliable one, but it is easy to do for yourself.

Causes

We'll be going into the common foods in more detail later in the book, and into how to identify and avoid them, but these are the top four prime suspects in food allergies. Because they crop up in

LOSS OF INSIGHT

Years ago, I was allergic to milk, and I probably had been for some time. I had figured it out and mostly stayed off dairy products. My dietitian at that time said, "If you're milk-allergic, you may be OK with double cream." Double cream is a dense, rich cream commonly used in desserts and other foods in Britain. The reason it may not cause a reaction is because most of the milk protein has been removed from it. So I agreed to test this out.

I had to drive past her house and I arranged to stop in for lunch. For dessert, she served a fruit crumble on which I poured double cream. Within minutes, I was walking around her kitchen trying to stay awake, but I didn't realize that was why. I even decided to get in the car and drive in order to clear my head! But it wasn't until I woke up in the wrong lane on the freeway for the second time that I somehow figured through the brain fog that this might not be a great idea. I pulled over into a service station and fell asleep on the steering wheel for half an hour. Then, finally, the message got through to me! I called her up and said, "I nearly died of double cream just now."

When your brain is a target organ for an allergy, of course you don't think straight. You lose insight, you lose mental processing power. Also, because you lose memory function, you often need to write things down.

so many foods, it is easy to be taking wheat or dairy products several times a day without realizing it. This can make it harder to spot the connection to your symptoms—it's not as straightforward as "every time I walk past a field of the stuff I start to sneeze." You will probably have to cut them out of your diet to see if you improve.

Wheat

Wheat is "the staff of life," which means the staple food on which we almost all depend in this society (in other cultures, of course, the staple is rice, potatoes, or yams). Wheat is not only the main ingredient of bread, pasta, and beer, but is also present in hidden form in many prepared and processed foods. Terms like "food starch" and "hydrolyzed vegetable protein" on the label may indicate the presence of wheat in a food. If you buy your lunch or snacks ready-made, the chances are they contain wheat.

Dairy

Milk and milk products are just as common in prepared foods as wheat. So as well as the obvious milk on your cereal, in your coffee or tea, in ice cream or yogurt, and of course in cheese, you also need to watch out for labels that list ingredients such as "lactose," "whey solids," or "caseinates."

Eggs

It is easy to spot the eggs in your diet and to stop eating them. But chicken eggs or parts of them, such as the egg white, are used to give smoothness to liquid foods like mayonnaise, salad dressing, and ice cream, and in baked foods such as cakes and cookies, both to bind the food together and to glaze the top to make it shiny.

Additives

Additives are widely used to color food, to preserve it, and to boost the taste. If you prepare a meal yourself with foods as they came out of the ground or from the animal, then you can be sure there are no additives in it. Otherwise, you can't—if you buy a food in a packet or box, then someone has had a chance to add chemical additives, and while these should be declared on the label, it can feel like it takes a degree in food science to interpret these.

CHEMICAL SENSITIVITIES

Chemical sensitivities refers to sensitivity to chemical fumes, not chemicals present in foods, which are dealt with under food allergies and intolerances. Fumes are small molecules that can be carried on airborne particles such as pollen and pollution, in water vapor, and just in the air as a scent or smell. They get straight to the mucous membranes of your nose, mouth, and throat, where they can both set off local immune reactions (producing familiar symptoms such as rhinitis, coughing, and wheezing) and also trigger the nervous system to cause headaches, migraines, symptoms of anxiety or panic, and even blackouts. There are recorded cases of fumes triggering anaphylaxis (a severe systemic reaction that can sometimes prove fatal). So the portal of entry for fumes is the same as for pollens—the upper respiratory system—but there is more than one mechanism happening. The reactions in the nervous system tend to produce immediate symptoms, so they are more evident and it is easier to identify the triggers, but the immune reactions can be delayed by hours, and so they are harder to spot and deal with. The immune reactions are also likely to be set off by other triggers, such as foods.

Symptoms

Burning—Perhaps the most common symptom is burning and/or soreness of the nose and throat on inhaling fumes. This can happen with a very small amount of the fume, and it typically comes on instantaneously.

Cough—In some cases, the burning and inflammation of the

mucous membranes will set off a dry cough, which can also be immediate.

Rhinitis, wheezing—As with inhalants like pollens, chemical fumes can set off the mechanisms that the body uses to try to expel what it identifies as undesirable. Because these responses work through the immune system, they may not be immediate, and in fact can take up to twenty-four hours to show.

Headache, migraine—These symptoms are probably nervous system symptoms, but we're not sure. They can be immediate or delayed. In a 1983 study at the Great Ormond Street Children's Hospital in London, 25 percent of children with migraine got them in reaction to fumes; all of the children reacted with migraine to foods as well.[2]

Anxiety, hyperventilation—Also direct physical effects on the nervous system, these symptoms are normally immediate, and they provide some useful insight into the mechanisms involved (see inset "Alarm Responses").

Smell sensitivity—Many, maybe most, people with chemical sensitivities report that they are very sensitive to the smell of the fumes. That is to say, the chemicals that would give them symptoms at a much lower dose than the rest of us, they can detect the smell of those chemicals at an even lower dose. This is pretty useful, allowing them to take early avoiding action. I have one patient with fume sensitivity who lost her sense of smell for an unrelated reason, and it made things much worse for her. She never knew she had been exposed until she started to get a headache and other symptoms.

Causes

Most of the chemicals setting off these reactions are synthetic and/or petrochemical-derived, but not all. Rapeseed—that bright yellow-flowered crop that you sometimes see big stretches of from

ALARM RESPONSES

Smells can be remarkably powerful in bringing back memories, especially the emotional content, the feeling, that goes with the memory. This can happen because there are direct connections from the olfactory nerves in the nose to the limbic system. Deep inside the brain, the limbic system dates from well back in evolution, and its earliest function may have been to enable an animal to respond rapidly to the smell of a predator by activating the whole nervous system in order to run away. In humans, it is involved with appetites such as hunger and sex, with addiction, and with motivation and goal-oriented actions. It has a lot to do with how we handle stresses and challenges in life.

Decades ago, psychiatrists sometimes treated severely emotionally disturbed people with an operation called a frontal lobotomy, which cut the nerves from the limbic system to the prefrontal cortex, the "thinking brain." This tended to leave them passive, unmotivated, and generally uninterested in anything.

So the limbic system is primitive and basic, and it's involved in emotional and instinctive responses. It is too deep in the "old brain" to respond to conscious commands, but it can drive our actions without us realizing it. And it can be triggered straight from the nose. In fact, it is the reason women wear perfume and men wear cologne.

This explains how a nervous system reaction to fumes can develop, but not why. Two facts can help us here. The first is that the typical story of chemical fume sensitivity is that the person was once heavily exposed to one chemical, got ill, and afterward got symptoms from exposure to just a tiny amount of it. Later, they also reacted to exposure to an increasing number of other chemicals as well, all at ultra-low doses. Some scientists have called this process TILT (toxin-induced loss of tolerance), because the initial event is as much a toxic event as an allergic one. In fact, it's probably both of the following factors:

- A big dose of something to which both the immune system and the nervous system are capable of becoming sensitized and reacting.

- A big enough dose of a toxin, exactly the same molecule, to overload our detoxifying mechanisms, build up to a high level in the body, and so poison our immune and/or nervous systems for long enough to cause them to respond badly.

The second fact, uncovered in a 2004 paper from Canada,[3] is that having certain combinations of genes known to lead to a build-up of toxins in the body can greatly increase your risk of developing chemical sensitivities. So if your body is genetically programmed to be not very good at removing toxins, they are more likely to build up and trigger an event like TILT.

When this happens, a direct link has been established from the smell receptors in your nose to the limbic system, bypassing conscious control and activating your "fight-or-flight" responses by releasing epinephrine, which alerts/arouses/alarms you. This reflex widens the eyes so you see better, increases blood flow to muscles, raises heart and breathing rates—all hard-wired animal survival mechanisms. Increasing breathing rate is necessary to increase oxygen intake for the anticipated burst of activity; now that we are no longer hunter-gatherers, that burst hardly ever comes, but we have not lost the reflex. The result is that newly programmed stresses such as chemical exposures can cause you to hyperventilate involuntarily. It can also lead some doctors to write you off as a head case—indeed, to write the whole of chemical sensitivity off as being psychological. Don't let them.

your airliner window seat—produces large quantities of volatile compounds that can set off this kind of reaction. Similar molecules occur in many essential oils and in perfumes. But the large majority of chemicals capable of setting off fume reactions fall into the group known as terpenes.

Terpenes (the word does come from the same root as turpentine) are fundamental molecules that form the building blocks for a lot of other molecules, including the steroid hormones on which we all depend. But a lot of plants produce simple terpenes; they have been found to have natural pesticide activity, which is probably one reason plants make them, and they also produce some familiar smells. The odors of lemon and of pine, for instance, are terpenes. In fact, the plants that produce the most terpenes are the conifers, and the fossil fuels that we pump out of the ground are predominantly compressed out of buried forests of conifers. The molecule that gives you that real lemon scent from lemons is closely related to the molecule that gives you the synthetic lemon scent from your toilet cleaner and similar to the molecules coming out of that car exhaust. And because some of them are smells, your nose has receptors shaped to accept just this kind of molecule and send a signal to the brain.

Exhaust Fumes

The burnt petrochemicals coming out the back of most automobiles, not to mention airplanes and trains, are triggers for most fume-sensitive people.

Tobacco Smoke

Other people's smoke can easily set off reactions.

Perfumes and Scents

Although some people react only to specific perfumes, most have a problem with them all.

Cleaning fluids, Disinfectants, Household Chemicals

Those bottles you store under the kitchen sink are common triggers, with or without added scent.

Aerosols and Air Fresheners

There is now a growing amount of evidence linking these chemicals

THE DOMINO EFFECT
OF CHEMICAL SENSITIVITY

Chris is a computer nerd. He was always a keen cyclist, and one day he slip-streamed behind a pretty smelly, polluting truck for a couple of miles, right in the cloud of burnt diesel exhaust. He had to give up when the fumes made him feel dizzy, weird, and ill. He got over that within hours, but a few days later noticed that just cycling down a city street made him ill. Then it was chemicals coming off the computers at work, then toner fumes from the photocopier, then his wife's perfume.

not only to fume reactions but, according to a survey in Bristol, England, to diarrhea and ear ache in infants and to headache and depression in their mothers.[4] We don't yet know the mechanism for this, but the link seems real.

Solvents, Adhesives, Newsprint

There are some startling reports of kids who play on new carpets and get nasty nervous system reactions, and all of these chemicals can trigger problems in sensitive people.

Alcohol

People with chemical sensitivities usually find that just a half-glass of white wine, for instance, will make them high and give them a real hangover. Maybe the chemicals overload the liver and make it difficult to process alcohol in the usual way? Anyway, it is a useful confirmation of a chemical problem.

DIAGNOSING ALLERGIES

Doctors are often inclined to think that diagnosing illness is their job, and that patients shouldn't worry their little heads about it.

Sometimes they have a point—doctors are in a much better position to diagnose cancer, for instance, because they have the expertise, the laboratories. and the diagnostic machines. But with allergies/intolerances/sensitivities, there are a couple of problems.

The first is that it takes a long time to change the consensus in medicine, rather like turning around a supertanker on the high seas. It took about twenty years for medicine to accept that food intolerances were real and important, and it's likely to take that long again to accept that chemical sensitivities are real. And during that time, allergies are getting more common and more serious. So you may just have to get on with it yourself.

The second is that, for some doctors, a diagnosis just means giving the symptoms a name—allergic rhinitis, for instance. But that is not much help to you without identifying the causes. All the doctor can do is offer you drugs to control the symptoms, and all you can do is keep going back for more pills. For me, a diagnosis of allergic rhinitis is only complete when it identifies the allergens, the triggers that set it off. Only then can you start to take control of it yourself.

CHAPTER 2

ALLERGIES THAT KILL

We are in an allergy epidemic all across the developed world. However you measure it, rates of allergy have risen massively over the past three decades. And some of these allergies can be fatal—namely, anaphylaxis, asthma, and oral allergy syndrome.

The fastest-growing type of allergy is anaphylaxis, with asthma not far behind. Hospital admissions for anaphylaxis have risen alarmingly in the past decade alone. In the United States, there are more than 60,000 cases of anaphylaxis every year; about 300 of those cases are fatal. Asthma rates have been climbing in the same way, and the prevalence in the U.S. is now estimated at about 11 percent, meaning that one person in nine suffers from asthma at some time. Every year, more than 5,000 people die from it. Both diagnoses have increased the fastest in young children.

Oral allergy syndrome is something we haven't known about for very long. It has also been called oral anaphylaxis, oral hay fever, and the pollen-food allergy syndrome, which tells you how it happens—it is a cross-reaction that develops between specific pollens and specific foods. Exposure to either can then give immediate symptoms of itching and swelling at the point of contact, such as the lips, tongue, mouth, even the throat. It can be mild and harmless, but can also be so severe that it merges into anaphylaxis.

All three diagnoses are true allergies by anybody's standards. They involve increases in the immunoglobulin E (IgE) antibody class, which can often be picked up in blood tests. They can all be dangerous, so we'll treat them together here. They all tend to merge into each other—severe asthma can become anaphylaxis, and indeed it can be hard to decide which is which. Oral allergy syndrome can become anaphylaxis as well. Since these allergic reactions can be life-threatening, it is important to know how to recognize them and what to do about them. It is important to know what to do in an acute emergency, as well as how to reduce your risk in the long-term.

ANAPHYLAXIS

The main event in both anaphylaxis and asthma is simple, all due to the release of histamine. This is what you take antihistamines for when seeking relief from a lesser, more local allergy, but in these two diagnoses the histamine release is more widespread and more dangerous. Histamine makes the blood capillaries more porous (leaky), allowing both fluid and blood cells to get out into the tissues and produce inflammation, which is necessary to counteract infections and repair damage. Histamine is also necessary for the production of acid in the stomach, so we all need it. But in anaphylaxis, so much histamine is released all through the body that it causes widespread swelling, including in the lungs, and so much fluid gets out during this swelling that the blood volume, and therefore the blood pressure, can drop dangerously. The only real antidote is epinephrine (adrenaline), which constricts the capillaries and stops them from leaking.

Symptoms

Inflammation—The main symptom, which almost everyone experiences, is inflammation of the epithelial surfaces of the body (the skin and the mucous membranes). On the skin, this may manifest as a general flushing or as urticaria (hives or nettle rash; raised red blobs of any shape and size). On the mucous membranes, inflammation can be more dramatic, with angioedema (severe swelling of the lips, tongue, and/or eyes). This can also happen in the throat, causing hoarseness of the voice and harsh, difficult breathing (stridor). It can cause a blocked and/or runny nose and sneezing. In the lungs, of course, it can constrict the bronchial tubes and cause wheezing or asthma.

Hypotension—The loss of blood volume into the tissues can cause a drop in blood pressure, and if severe, this can amount to circulatory collapse. Be sure that you don't stand up in this situation—this will make it worse. You may feel light-headed and even black out. The pulse will race and may go irregular, and you may feel chest pain from the strain on the heart.

Other symptoms—You may experience stomach cramps, diarrhea, and/or vomiting as the gut becomes inflamed. You may feel a sense of panic or of impending doom.

Symptoms in Children

It is important to be able to spot anaphylaxis in a small child, because they can't tell you what is happening to them. If a child is already allergic, you need to be aware of the possibility of anaphylactic shock, but some anaphylaxis events happen out of the blue, with no previous allergy problems. Look for these signs:

• Flushing or swelling (of the skin, mouth, nose, throat, or eyes)

• Difficulty breathing

• Faintness

• Fast pulse

When in doubt, regard it as anaphylaxis and act accordingly (seek immediate medical care).

Causes

Anaphylaxis is an allergic reaction, and in 80 percent of cases the probable cause can be identified; the rest are known by doctors as idiopathic (of unknown origin). But whether it is a food, a wasp sting, or a drug that causes it, you may not have come into contact with it before (at least to your knowledge).

Foods

The most common causes are nuts, milk and dairy products, eggs, and seafood and fish. Usually, but not always, there has been some kind of mild allergic reaction to it before. The big exception to this is nut (particularly peanut) reactions in children (see box "Peanuts"). Typically, it takes around thirty minutes from eating (or even touching) the food to when the symptoms start.

Stings

Wasps, yellow-jackets, and bees can all sting you and set off an anaphylactic reaction. Two-thirds of people who get this reaction have never known a severe reaction to a sting before. Average time from sting to symptoms is fifteen minutes.

Drugs

The biggest single drug-related cause of anaphylaxis is penicillin, but other antibiotics can cause it as well. Aspirin and the other nonsteroidal, anti-inflammatory drugs (NSAIDs, such as ibuprofen) probably come next in frequency, but any drug can potentially be a culprit. So can anesthetics, muscle relaxants, and the contrast media used in x-rays. Of course, reactions to these will normally happen in a hospital, where all the necessary treatments will be at hand, but there is still no way to predict a reaction. Eighty percent of people who get drug-induced anaphylaxis have never had a reaction to it before. The reaction time is fast, averaging five minutes from drug to symptoms.

Desensitization

Shots for allergies can also set off anaphylaxis—at least the "incremental" desensitizing shots used by most hospital allergists can. That's why they should only ever be given in a hospital or clinic setting, where the necessary treatments are available.

PEANUTS

When cases of anaphylaxis were tracked down to a food, the most common single trigger has been peanuts.[1] This reaction has been happening more and more in younger and younger children. What puzzled scientists for some time is that many of these kids had never been given a peanut before in their life. There didn't seem to be a link to their mothers either eating peanuts or being allergic to them, so what was going on? The answer now seems to be that the kids had been exposed to peanut before, but not by mouth—they had touched them.

This can happen in two ways. The first is that there may be tiny particles (and they can be invisibly small) in the dust in our homes, tucked into the carpets or furniture. When babies start to crawl, they can come into contact with these particles. Of course, anaphylaxis happens more in people with a pre-existing allergic disease, and if your baby has eczema, the skin is inflamed and much more porous, letting the nut allergen into the system more easily.

The second way is by creams and lotions. The Avon Study in the United Kingdom discovered that using cream or lotion containing arachis oil (which is just another name for peanut oil) on skin with eczema was a major risk factor for developing peanut allergy, including anaphylaxis.[2] It can happen without any eczema as well. There is also the problem of soy, which contains allergens that are almost identical to the ones in peanuts. So, if you become allergic to soy, you may cross-react to peanuts, and vice versa. And there are a lot of oils, lotions, shampoos, and other products that contain soy oil. This means that you probably shouldn't use oils or lotions containing either peanut/arachis or soy oil on your baby.

This has also thrown out our advice on infant feeding. We used to think that you should take it slow in introducing new foods to your baby, but it now seems that it is better for them to eat a food first rather than to touch it first, so maybe we should give them little bits of lots of different foods from weaning onward. Of course, it doesn't change the fact that breastfeeding is best, and you should only breastfeed your baby for the first three to six months.

The desensitizing methods that I recommend elsewhere in this book have never, to my knowledge, been linked to anaphylaxis. That doesn't mean it couldn't happen; in twenty-five years of using enzyme-potentiated desensitization (EPD), I have just once become worried enough about a patient to draw up the epinephrine in case I needed it. In the end, I didn't. But the same precautions apply—EPD should be used only in a clinic setting where the antidotes are available, at least at first. After a few shots in this way, there should be no evidence of reactions suddenly occurring, and of course they should be working to make the allergy better.

Latex

For the last twenty years, medical staff and others have been using surgical gloves a lot more. This started with the human immunodeficiency virus (HIV) epidemic and has never gone away. To begin with, the gloves were made of latex (rubber), but now more people are switching to nonlatex gloves. The reason is an explosion of latex allergy in medical personnel, particularly operating room staff. The reaction doesn't have to be anaphylactic, but it often is. The other group who have been at high risk are babies born with spina bifida (neural tube defect). In this condition, the bottom of the spine can be open to the outside because it has not developed properly. Like the broken skin of eczema, it can lead to allergy when the baby is exposed to something by that route—in this case, to the latex from gloves. The frequency of reactions is slowing now in both groups, but there are still a lot of people who are at risk.

What to Do for Anaphylaxis

1. Get to hospital or to a doctor immediately. You can't handle this one on your own. There, they will give epinephrine and everything else that is needed.

2. If you have had an anaphylactic reaction or a near-miss, you need to discuss with your doctors about whether to carry an epinephrine auto-injector. This is a device that enables you to

inject yourself intramuscularly, even through clothing. This could save your life. Even so, all it does is buy you time to get to a hospital. You will need to be shown how to use it, of course, and we now advise people to carry two injectors because they can occasionally malfunction. They have a short shelf-life, so they need to be renewed every year.

WARNING!

Anaphylactic reactions can be biphasic; that is, you develop a reaction, and you treat it with epinephrine and it goes away, only to return minutes or hours (even a couple of days) later. So don't take chances—even if the epinephrine works, it doesn't mean you can just carry on as before. Get to a hospital anyway.

There is no vitamin cure or natural treatment in an acute anaphylactic reaction—you need immediate medical care. In the long run, though, you can do a number of things to reduce your risk, and this is dealt with, along with other allergies, later in this book. The first-line treatments are the essential anaphylaxis precautions recommended by your doctor.

ASTHMA

Although it is very complicated, involving a lot of different biochemicals and cells, asthma is an IgE reaction just the same as anaphylaxis, and it can be as dangerous. The majority of asthma cases (between 50 and 75 percent) can be tracked down to an allergic reaction. Most commonly, this is to something inhaled (because it is the portal of entry), but it can also be to a food, a drug, or even an infection.

When asthma is only mild and infrequent, you can treat it with the measures for allergies in general, described elsewhere in this book. You always need to be working with a doctor, however severe your asthma is, and to listen to what he or she says, but you do have a right to form your own opinion about treatment. Don't ignore your doctor's recommendations; rather, question and discuss them. This section is about serious asthma, when you may not have a choice about what to do.

Symptoms

Wheezing—This is the sole core symptom of asthma. Swelling of the mucous membranes of the airways reduces their bore-size because the lung cannot expand outward, being held by the ribcage. It means that breathing needs more effort, which is worse on the out-breath when you are applying pressure to the lungs to push the air out, which further constricts the tubes (bronchi). This is not without purpose—the air going through the narrower bronchi has to travel faster, which makes it more likely to push allergens, infecting organisms, and the mucus that develops around them out of the lungs. So, constriction of the bronchi can be viewed as an appropriate response to some factors, but it can still be too much of a response, and to the wrong things.

Cough—Coughing serves the same purpose as bronchoconstriction, to expel stuff from the bronchi. It can happen at the same time, and occasional attacks of asthma can easily be misdiagnosed as recurrent viral coughs.

Other symptoms—Asthma sufferers can often get other allergy problems, although it is more often the other way round: 60 percent of hay fever sufferers can get asthma when their hay fever is severe, for example. Unsurprisingly, asthma can also make you feel tired and unwell, and it can make the chest and shoulder muscles ache.

Causes

Asthma has always been divided into extrinsic and intrinsic types, meaning that the extrinsic is due to allergens that are inhaled, and the intrinsic has a nonallergic cause. But that is probably not true; yes, extrinsic allergy is usually due to a reaction to inhaled allergens, but it was called "extrinsic" simply because it was easier to recognize an inhaled reaction. It is also an IgE reaction or classic allergy. Intrinsic asthma, on the other hand, is probably due in most cases to non-inhalant reactions: allergies/intolerances/sensitivities to foods, chemical fumes, and bacteria, and quite often to aspirin and other NSAIDs. IgE levels are low, and it is not an IgE reaction. But the strongest evidence that it is an allergic (in the broad sense) reaction is that it usually responds to desensitization.

WARNING!

If an asthma reaction to a non-inhalant is immediate, happening in less than an hour, it may be heading toward anaphylaxis. Act accordingly and seek immediate medical attention.

What to Do Immediately

See the rest of this book for how to deal with asthma in the long-term. This section is only about treatment of an acute episode.[4]
Could this be anaphylaxis? If so:

- **Don't** stand up.

- **Do** get to hospital.

If you have epinephrine, it must be for a reason, so use it if in any doubt.
Otherwise, use a bronchodilator drug (an inhaler) if you have it. Nebulizers are better at getting the drug into a constricted lung than plain inhalers. Steroid inhalers take around eighteen hours to work, so don't bother, and definitely don't depend on them. The hospital can give you steroids by injection if needed.

Inhalant Allergens

All the allergens listed under inhalant allergies in Chapter 1 may cause asthma. Reactions are usually "immediate" in onset (within minutes) and short-lived, although a minority of asthma sufferers get a reaction that takes 12–18 hours to begin and lasts up to a week. If this happens in pollen season, it means you will wheeze for the whole season, as you are repeatedly exposed.

Foods

Milk and dairy products, eggs, food additives, and nuts are the most common causes. There is no reason to suppose that any given food is unable to cause this reaction, however. The reaction is typically delayed by at least an hour, and possibly by up to four days, and it can last for days as well.

Chemical Fumes

Perfumes, tobacco smoke, exhaust or petrol fumes, cleaning fluids, and household chemicals are the primary culprits. The reaction can be rapid or delayed.

Gut Bacteria and Yeasts

Overgrowth of *Candida* and other yeast organisms is a real problem, but asthmatic reactions triggered by these organisms are not common. It is the bacteria in the gut that can set off asthma. One study found that a third of "intrinsic" asthma cases reacted to components of their gut flora and responded to appropriate antibiotics.[3] Because prescription medications are likely to be needed in the treatment of this problem, you should consult your doctor about this.

ORAL ALLERGY SYNDROME

Oral allergy syndrome has been called both "hay fever in the mouth" and "oral anaphylaxis," which tells you a lot about its wide range of severity. It's an allergic reaction, and it happens in the mouth and/or throat, but it can be just a faint itch or tingling (some people quite enjoy that), or your mouth and throat can swell up instantly, preventing you from breathing.

Symptoms

The symptoms of oral allergy syndrome can range from mild to severe.

Mild symptoms—Slight itching or tingling of the lips or tongue immediately after the food is touched to them (most reactions happen within five minutes, and all within thirty minutes).

Moderate symptoms—Itching/tingling and swelling where the food touches. If the food is swallowed, this can happen in the throat and even further down in the airway, and you may vomit.

Severe symptoms—Immediate severe swelling of the mouth and throat, which can interfere with breathing. It can also provoke general anaphylaxis if swallowed. The reaction can even be triggered by kissing someone who has recently eaten the food, and just smelling the food may cause itching of the nose and throat or even asthma. This type of reaction is seen in no more than 3 percent of cases.

Causes

It is usually not difficult to discover the cause when a food causes immediate symptoms, so most sufferers know which foods give them oral allergy syndrome. But there are some recognized cross-reactions that cause the large majority of oral allergy syndrome cases, so it is worth knowing about them. This is not definitive though; opinions do vary on exactly which foods cross-react, and we are learning more about it all the time. There are some foods—maybe many—which can cause the oral symptoms without there being any cross-reaction to a pollen. Also, cooking the food may or may not abolish or reduce the reaction.

These are the known cross-reactions[5]:

- Ragweed pollen with banana, melon, watermelon, zucchini—people with common hay fever due to ragweed may cross-react to these foods.

- Birch pollen with apple, apricot, carrot, celery, cherry, kiwi, melon, nectarine, peach, peanut, potato, tomato—it is thought that around 70 percent of people with birch allergy also have oral allergy syndrome.

- Latex with avocado, banana, fig, passion fruit, celery, citrus, kiwi, tomato, grape, papaya, peanut, pineapple—see the anaphylaxis section above for more information on latex allergy.

What to Do

- If severe, oral allergy syndrome may require epinephrine treatment.
- Milder forms will often respond to antihistamines.

Once you have identified an oral reaction to a food, you should avoid it. It is probably wise to avoid all the other cross-reacting foods listed above to stop from developing a reaction and to reduce an existing one.

To check for an allergic reaction, try simply smelling the food. If you don't get a reaction to the smell, you can check by just touching it briefly to the lips or tongue—any resulting swelling there is unlikely to be serious.

Desensitization can help (see later in this book for more information). In a severe reaction, it can reduce the severity; in a mild reation, it may enable you to eat the food without symptoms. Be warned, though, that a negative tongue test for a particular food—no tingling or swelling when you touch the food to your tongue—is *not* a guarantee that it is safe for you to eat.

CHAPTER 3

AVOIDING INHALANTS

So, you think you may have an allergy? What can you do about it? This chapter is about the obvious first step—staying away from it (avoiding) and/or cutting it out of your life and environment (removing). These are two aspects of the same thing, which you want to do in order to confirm or refute your diagnosis and to stay well (or at least less unwell).

There are limits to how much you can do to avoid and remove allergens. If you have hay fever from ragweed pollen, for instance, only relocating to the Arctic Circle will really work, and even that's not guaranteed. You will find that there are limits to how much you are prepared to do as well, to how much your life will allow you to do. It is difficult to avoid wheat or dairy products totally if you want to have a life outside your home. But there are also steps you can take to protect yourself as well, which we will discuss later in the book. In this chapter and the following one, we'll look at avoiding and removing allergens, both for diagnosis and for treatment.

Reactions to inhalants are usually the easiest to figure out, because they tend to be a direct cause-and-effect reaction: you react when they are there, and you don't react when they aren't there. So, with a little bit of extra knowledge, you can usually get a positive identification on them. It may not be so easy to avoid and remove them, though, and that is where the strategies in this book may help.

POLLENS

The good news about pollens is that they are only around for part of the year; the bad news is that when they are around, it is just about impossible to avoid them. So, diagnosis is a matter of observing the pattern—when and where you get the symptoms—and applying some common sense. However, treatment can be trickier.

Ragweed

There are a whole list of weeds that can set off allergies with their pollen, but in North America the most important by far is ragweed. Around 75 percent of people with hay fever have a reaction to ragweed (most will have reactions to other pollens or inhalants as well). So, in a spirit of "know your enemy," here are some basics. Ragweed is a hardy beast: the seeds can lay dormant in the soil for years, and it thrives on waste ground, vacant lots, roadsides, river banks, and the edges of fields. No place in the United States is free of ragweed; in Canada, the two ends of the country, Newfoundland and most of British Columbia, are free of ragweed, but nowhere else is. It thrives in dry, sunny locations, which is why a vacant lot can be ideal for it.

The ragweed pollen season is from July to November at its longest, but it has a shorter season in many places; the peak time for pollen is usually around September. Warm air rises, and the ragweed plant has evolved to take advantage of that to spread its seed. So the pollen is around in the air you breathe mainly when the ground and air are warming up, from a couple of hours after sunrise through midafternoon. High humidity also encourages the release of pollen, so damp weather is worse for sufferers, but rain washes the pollen down to the ground again, reducing symptoms.

How can this information help? Well, it should allow you to confirm ragweed as a culprit in your allergies. If your sneezing and runny nose start midmorning and ease off in the evening and through the night, think of ragweed. And since almost all other pollens stop being released by the end of August, if your symptoms continue through to September or later, that points to ragweed as well. But remember that you will likely react to other pollens or to other allergens such as molds, and that their seasons may overlap.

For avoiding, though, I'm afraid there's not much help. You may be able to get out of the ragweed zone by going to the coast or into the mountains, but even that's not guaranteed. Things may be easier indoors, especially if there is an air-conditioning system with a HEPA filter (a high-efficiency particulate air filter should remove nearly all pollen, including ragweed), although you can't stay indoors all the time.

Other Weeds

That "whole list" of weeds I mentioned above includes sagebrush, plantain, and tumbleweed, each with their own season. The entire season for weed pollens in general extends from April through November in the Western states, and from May through September in the Northeast. The same facts apply, though, regarding outdoor versus indoor, warm versus cold, and so on, as mentioned above for ragweed. The same difficulties apply regarding avoidance as well.

MOLDS

Molds are strange things: they're not animals like us, but they're not plants either. They are multicelled organisms, but all the cells are the same and they can form into strings of cells called hyphae. Sometimes when you find mold growing on something in your refrigerator, you can just see a thatch of these tiny filaments. They reproduce by means of spores, which are their version of seeds, that are typically spread through the air, some using ingenious devices such as launch by the splash of raindrops. Molds can

THUNDERSTORMS AND ALLERGIES

We've always known that some hay fever and asthma sufferers experienced worse symptoms during thunderstorms, and some people only got symptoms during a storm. But we didn't quite know why. Then, on June 25, 1994, there was a dramatic thunderstorm over London, England. In the following thirty hours, 640 people attended emergency rooms across London with hay fever or asthma—this is around ten times the number of people that would be expected, even in midsummer. Professor Jean Emberlin, who runs the Pollen Research Unit at the University of Worcester, was in London that night. It took her several years, and the help of a range of climate scientists and others, to discover what happened that night, and what happens in other storms.[1]

You would imagine that in high summer the only allergen around was pollens, and that all those people must have been pollen-allergic. In fact, in most outbreaks of "thunderstorm asthma," the problem is a combination of pollens and molds plus high humidity and high electrical charge. There are molds that use the splash of raindrops to launch into the air. Pollen grains actually disappear from the air after thunderstorms, effectively washed away by the heavy rain. You've probably noticed how clean the air looks after a storm and how visibility improves— well, that's because the pollen has been washed to the ground.

But with the right combination of high humidity, warm air rising, and intense static electrical charge, which can happen before storms, pollen is released by plants and lifted up into the air. There they soak up water from the humid air and swell until they burst, releasing the much smaller granules within them, granules small enough to get right down into the lungs. Then, the molds—and one in particular called *Cladosporium*—get launched by the first raindrops and can also be carried up into the air by the powerful updrafts and electrical charge. The molds combine with the tiny pollen granules to form the virulent allergy cocktail that caused all those admissions.

> But this obviously doesn't happen with every thunderstorm; a complex combination of events is necessary for it all to come together. What can we learn from this? Mainly, that allergies are often more complicated than we think. You think that you only react to pollen, but it could be molds as well. And the pollen-sensitive asthmatic who is rushed to the hospital whenever the mowers come around is probably also responding to a cocktail of pollen and the mold *Cladosporium.*

produce three different types of illness: allergy, infection, and toxicity. We are mainly concerned with the first of these.

With some important exceptions, molds need a warm, humid environment to grow, which is why they can sometimes be the first sign that damp has gotten into your home. A study by indoor environment specialists at the Environmental Protection Agency (EPA) in 2007 calculated that about 47 percent of American homes have mold or damp problems.[2] Offices and other buildings are not much better. Air conditioning doesn't necessarily help because the mold can live right in the system and be spread around by it. The EPA also estimated that around 21 percent of asthma cases in the U.S. are caused by molds.

I worked on a small island in the Pacific years ago, and we were warned that leather would quickly go moldy there, which it did. All the houses had lightbulbs in the closet to dry it out, but it didn't really help—shoes and handbags still developed steadily growing patches of mold within weeks. When the island nation got its independence from Britain, the government sent out a retired general to organize the handover and celebrations. He complained that "You can't even buy a decent pair of shoes here, dash it!"—which was true, but he wasn't around long enough to find out why; they would have been moldy by the time he bought them.

Outdoor molds are mostly seasonal, but it is easy to be misled by them. They can be dramatic too: my sister told me that all her tomatoes were wiped out in a single night by tomato blight, along with all the neighbors' tomatoes; they woke to find all the plants covered in a brown-black dust. The source was probably plants that had been infected the previous year, and either left in the ground, composted, or just dumped. The correct advice is to burn infected plants, not leave them lying around.

There are many thousands of different molds, but here are some of the more common varieties.

Aspergillus—*Aspergillus* grows in rotting vegetation and in mattresses and animal bedding; there are high levels found in bird cages also. So, *Aspergillus* can be a problem both indoors and outdoors—mainly in the Autumn in temperate climates, but as you move into tropical climes, the more of the year it is present. One subtype, *Aspergillus niger,* is used in the manufacture of black tea, which means there is a cross-reaction possible between the mold and the tea (it is pretty uncommon though). In addition to allergies (mainly rhinitis and asthma), *Aspergillus* can cause a deep-seated infection in the lungs, especially if you have damaged or vulnerable lungs in the first place, including from asthma. You could have asthma, which leads to aspergillosis in the lungs, and this then causes more asthma and further damages the lungs. Treatment of this problem will require a combination of antifungal medication to kill the organism and additional treatment of the allergies.

Botrytis—The cause of the "noble rot," or the spontaneous fermentation of grapes that makes certain wines special, *Botrytis* grows as a grey film on many fruits and other plants. It can be around all summer, with high levels near blighted crops.

Cladosporium—*Cladosporium* grows on dying grass leaves, so peak season overlaps and extends after the grass pollen season. Maximum release of *Cladosporium* is in humid weather and at the start of thunderstorms by splash launch.

Sporobolomyces—Technically, *Sporobolomyces* is a yeast, a microscopic organism that grows on the underside of leaves and uses an amazing catapult mechanism to launch its spores, with an unbelievable acceleration of 25,000 Gs. This tends to happen in the evening of a sunny day as the humidity rises, which is why the classic pattern is of asthma coming on for no apparent reason in the middle of a barbecue.

Stachybotrys—See box "Toxic Mold" on the following page.

Ustilago—*Ustilago* grows as a blight on grain crops, and spores are released in the same conditions (sunny summer days) as are pollen grains. This can potentially confuse the diagnosis in hay fever.

We tend to think of molds as a problem in the Fall, during damp weather and in damp places, and this is broadly true, but there are so many exceptions that, in reality, mold reactions can happen any time of the year and anywhere. Avoidance is therefore a problem. Of course, indoor molds can be reduced by keeping the place dry and clean, and particularly by getting rid of any leaks and damp patches, but that still doesn't guarantee freedom from mold. The National Center for Healthy Housing (www.nchh.org) offers a wide range of advice and resources for tackling damp and other indoor problems.

Here are some basic steps you can take:

- Water leaks and drips—Get the whole plumbing system checked, at least yearly, for leaks and faulty seals or washers, and get them put right. Check gutters and down-pipes for blockages that may spill over and cause dampness on walls.

- Water damage—Check under the sink, behind the bath, behind the washer, and under the water heater or boiler for any signs of leaks, past or present. Fix the leaks *and* repair the damage.

- Damp—Dampness can get in, particularly through outside walls. Check in cupboards, behind cavity walls, and in roof spaces for any signs of damp, then cut it out and replace it.

TOXIC MOLD

There has been a lot of publicity in the last few years about toxic mold, mainly due to some high-profile legal cases. But while allergies to molds, with symptoms such as rhinitis, sinusitis, and asthma, are well-accepted, the idea that molds cause other symptoms, particularly neurological ones, anything more than rarely is controversial at least among scientists. There is evidence for this, however. Two studies of heavily mold-exposed patients (198 total) found that fatigue and weakness was present in 71 percent in one study, 100 percent in the other; bad memory, concentration difficulties, and other neuro-cognitive problems were found in 67 percent and 46 percent, respectively; bowel symptoms were seen in 58 percent and 25 percent.[3] Other studies show that exposed people do worse on tests of coordination, balance, reflex time, and visual acuity.[4]

The most common mold suspected in these problems is called *Stachybotrys*, which usually produces a black mold growth, though it can also be white or pink. It is known to release mycotoxins, poisons that can affect the nerves and the immune system. One of the mycotoxins, stachylysin, can cause hemorrhage, including the potentially fatal infant lung hemorrhage. Others, such as trichothecenes, can seriously affect the nervous and immune systems. Of course, immunocompromised people (with HIV, for instance) are particularly vulnerable, but allergies can mean that your immune system is malfunctioning and you are also more vulnerable.

Mold toxins are a suspect in causing sudden infant death syndrome (SIDS) or cot death.[5] What seems to happen is that the molds can react with chemicals such as flame retardants in the baby's mattress to produce highly toxic gases, which the baby breathes in. Simply having the baby sleep on his or her back, or wrapping the mattress up thoroughly so that the baby is not exposed to the toxic fumes, may help prevent cot deaths.

- Ventilation—Make sure that the whole house is reasonably ventilated, including the parts you can't see, like roof spaces and cavity walls.

DUST MITES

Looking like something out of the *Alien* movies (in miniature), dust mites are rather creepy little creatures that live off animal debris—including skin particles from us, fur particles from pets, feathers in pillows, and even wool. An adult human sheds as much as a pound of skin debris in a year, which is enough to feed up to a million dust mites. They like warmth and moisture, so the easiest way to get exposed to them is from your pillow; as you sleep, you breathe out warm, moist air, which encourages the mites to come out and party, right "in your face." The mites have only a very primitive digestive system, so they have to eat each particle of food several times, regurgitating it in between with their digestive enzymes in it, and it is these particles that are most allergenic.

On account of their lifestyle, your maximum exposure to dust mites is usually in bed at night; even though they are all over your house, you probably don't stick your nose in them anywhere else. So, the typical pattern for dust mite allergy is of symptoms (blocked nose, sneezing, coughing, wheezing, and itchy eyes) building up through the night to a peak when you wake up. This may or may not disturb your sleep, and if it doesn't, it is easy to misread the situation and think that the symptoms only happen when you wake up and get up. When people tell me they only sneeze first thing in the morning and it's gone in an hour or so, chances are it is dust mites they are reacting to.

There is one completely safe method that you might like to try first, which is killing the mites by freezing. Put your pillow in a clean garbage bag, and use a vacuum cleaner to suck out all the air, making it as small as possible. Then, tie it up and put it in the freezer for twenty-four hours. Take it out, open it, and shake it up well in the bag—this should leave a small amount of dust at the bottom of the bag. Vacuum it all over and put it back on the bed. You can do the same for stuffed toys, like a teddy bear, if your child likes to have it close at night. If this helps, you can repeat it as often as you like.

If it doesn't help, you probably have to tackle the rest of the bedding or even carpets, and those you can't freeze so easily. There are special covers for bedding that don't let the mites through, and these are often helpful; many websites and department stores offer them. There are also sprays you can get for bedding that kill off the mites as well as other airborne allergens such as molds; non-toxic, eco-friendly ones use alcohol and enzymes to break down the proteins and kill the mites. They generally help, for a few weeks or months anyway. I wouldn't recommend frequent use of a spray based on potentially toxic chemicals, but the eco-friendly sprays should be safe.

DEAD FLY DUST

Dust mites and their food particles are the major allergen in house dust, but there is one more that can be important—dead flies. Gross, I know, but the corpses of flies can gradually break up and linger as dust, particularly in places that you don't clean often—garages, attics, closets, and workshops, for instance. They can cause the same allergies (rhinitis, asthma) as dust mites, but with a different pattern. The symptoms typically happen on sweeping up in places like the garage, but *don't* happen in bed at night. Thorough cleaning is the only way to reduce your exposure.

ANIMALS

Just about any animal that has fur or feathers can cause allergies; this is usually pretty obvious, but we should say a few words about cats. It has been shown that cats make a protein called Fel (for feline) d1, which seems to be the main cause of cat allergies. It is secreted in their saliva, so it gets onto their fur and from there it gets onto skin, clothing, and furnishings; it is very "sticky," which makes it very difficult to avoid. If the cat sleeps on the bed, then frequent washing of the bedding should help, and some people think that frequent washing of the cat does too. It is also one reason why little scratches and bites from a cat can produce so much inflammation (but bacteria are another reason, and they can be more dangerous and may need antibiotic treatment).

One interesting note is that if your immune system reacts to cats, it may still be able to learn to tolerate your own cat. It is unpredictable: heavy exposure to a cat (as to any other allergen) may also make things worse rather than better, but plenty of people have found that when a cat arrives in the home, they react to it for a while and then just stop. However, their reaction to other peoples' cats, and to cats in general, is likely to stay the same.

With all allergies to animals, staying away from them is the only real way to avoid exposure.

CHAPTER 4

AVOIDING FOODS AND CHEMICALS

In the last chapter, we looked at ways to avoid and remove inhalants in order to alleviate allergies. In this chapter, we will discuss similar strategies for food allergies/intolerances and chemical sensitivities.

FOOD ALLERGIES AND INTOLERANCES

With a certain amount of observation and logic, you may well be able to figure out which foods cause you to have an allergic reaction, although there are some pitfalls you need to be aware of, and sometimes you just can't do it without expert help. Two big caveats, however:

1. Food *allergies* can be severe and dangerous—for example, the growing number of peanut allergies may cause serious symptoms—so re-read Chapter 2: Allergies That Kill. If your allergies cause similar problems, follow the precautions.

2. Food *intolerances* are not so dangerous, but they are not so quick either. With an allergy, you usually react within an hour of exposure, but intolerances can easily take seventy-two hours to show (in rare cases, as much as a week). Factor in that a food can take forty-eight hours to pass through your digestive system, and it can be very hard to link a reaction to a particular food exposure. Often, the symptoms are just there all the time, or on a daily basis.

The Usual Suspects

The most common foods to cause reactions—the big five—are wheat, dairy, corn, food additives and colorings, and eggs. The reason may be that they are hidden in so many foods.

Wheat

Wheat is found in breads and cereals, as well as in cookie and pastries, pasta, and beer. Check the ingredients label on any prepared food for items such as "food starch" and "hydrolyzed vegetable protein," which also mean wheat.

Dairy

Milk and butter are the main types of dairy in the diet, along with cheeses (or something with cheese flavor). But dairy products are also hidden in many processed foods: watch out for "lactose," "whey solids," and "caseinates" on food labels.

WHEAT INTOLERANCE AND CELIAC DISEASE

There are two distinct disorders with wheat and it is possible to suffer from both. Wheat intolerance means that your immune system has been triggered to produce antibodies against wheat protein, and you are liable to get symptoms whenever you eat it. So long as you avoid wheat, you should be fine. Celiac syndrome (gluten enteropathy) is an autoimmune disease; that is, your immune system develops a reaction against your own tissues, in this case against the cells lining your bowel. To be precise, you develop a reaction to the combination of your cells with the gluten molecule in wheat.

Celiac can only happen if you have a particular "tissue-type" known as HLA-DQ2 or HLA-DQ8. *HLA* stands for human lymphocyte antigen, a family of proteins most easily found on

Lactose is a sugar, not a protein; and lactose intolerance is not an allergy—it is caused by lack of the enzyme lactase, which digests the sugar lactose. All mammals are born with this enzyme so they can breastfeed, but it is normally "switched off" after weaning. This is so for most humans too, but about 10,000 years ago those humans who moved into Northern Europe also took up farming and milking animals. They were healthier if they were able to keep the production of this enzyme switched on. Now, the descendants of those humans have spread around the world, taking this genetic "mutation" with them. In North America, people of European origin mostly have the new gene, while Native Americans and those of Afro-Caribbean origin mostly do not. This is evolution in operation, and the most obvious example of the genomics discussed in the next chapter.

If you have lactose intolerance, drinking milk or eating dairy products will give you symptoms such as abdominal bloating,

lymphocytes (white blood cells). Thirty percent of people have these types of HLA proteins, but still only a small percentage of them develop celiac disease. Doctors used to think that you had either full-on celiac, a severe disease affecting less than 1 percent of people, or you didn't have celiac at all, but we now realize that a lot of people have mild or partial celiac.

The effect of celiac is to produce atrophy (wasting away) of the villi, the tiny fingers lining the small bowel. This means a smaller surface area in the bowel so that you can't absorb nutrients from your food as well. That's why celiac sufferers get fatigue as a main symptom, along with bowel upsets. The bowel also becomes more "leaky," and food molecules can get through and attract the attention of the immune system. This leads to food intolerances, typically to wheat, but it can lead to other intolerances as well. Diagnosis is by a blood test for antibodies and treatment is a gluten-free diet for life.

wind, discomfort, and loose bowels. That's a black-and-white statement, but the reality is actually murkier: many lactose-intolerant people can manage a little milk or dairy products without symptoms, and many people get the same symptoms for different reasons such as irritable bowel syndrome. But if you get those particular symptoms, and if they are worse after eating or drinking milk products, then it's highly likely that you have lactose intolerance.

Corn (Maize)

Popcorn, cornflakes, hominy, and grits all contain corn. And Mexican food depends on corn to make tortillas, tamales, and many other foods. But corn seems to be just about omnipresent in processed foods, mainly as high-fructose corn syrup, which is used to sweeten most soft drinks, bakery goods, and jams and jellies, and is put in canned fruits, ketchup, even some dairy products. Bourbon is traditionally fermented from corn, Chinese food uses it as a staple ingredient, and when you lick a stamp or envelope there's corn starch in the adhesive.

Food Additives and Colorings

In Europe, these additives are known as "E numbers" after the numbering and classification system imposed by the Codex Alimentarius committee. Food labels can just state E102 (for tartrazine, one of the most problematic additives), not the full name. This hasn't happened in the U.S. yet, although it is increasingly common in Canada. It will happen eventually. There are several hundred chemicals that can be added to foods and drinks, in order to preserve it, flavor it, color it, or make it look better. Some are naturally occurring substances—even vitamin C has an E number—but some are petrochemicals and can cause problems, both toxicity (poisoning) and allergies. The food writer Michael Pollan once advised, "Don't eat foods that contain anything unpronounceable."[1] That covers most additives.

Eggs

Eggs show up in a long list of sauces, ice creams, bakery goods, and so on. It is not that eggs are bad for us—they are a great food, and you don't need to worry about the cholesterol content either. It is the fact that they are hidden in so many processed foods, so we eat them so often without knowing it that it puts them in the top five food allergies.

What to Do

Here's a simple plan for identifying and dealing with suspected food intolerances.

Keep a Food Diary

You may need a food diary to assist in your detective work. A food diary is a simple thing, but it has to be done with care. It consists of a record of what you eat and how you feel. Take a page for each day and write down *everything* you eat. Here's an example:

On waking: Grapefruit juice

Breakfast: Scrambled eggs, toast, marmalade, tea

Morning: Coffee

Lunch: Quiche (tomato, spinach), water

Next (you can do this later), you need to analyze it for hidden foods, the things that are present everywhere in our diet, especially in the processed foods you buy. Let's mark up this list for milk and dairy products, by underlining the foods that contain them:

On waking: Grapefruit juice

Breakfast: <u>Scrambled eggs</u>, <u>toast</u>, marmalade, tea

Morning: Coffee

Lunch: <u>Quiche</u> (tomato, spinach), water

The scrambled eggs were made with a little milk, there was butter on the toast, and milk in the tea. The quiche at lunch contained both milk and cheese. So only halfway through the day and this person already had consumed dairy products four times.

Keep a diary like the one above for a week. As well as everything you eat, note when you get symptoms. If you only get symptoms occasionally during the week, look back just over twenty-four hours from when the symptoms started—the food trigger is probably in that time frame. If you had bacon, say, or tuna, preceding the time you got symptoms and at no other time, you've got a prime suspect.

If that doesn't work, or if your symptoms happen every day, analyze the diary for wheat, dairy, and so on. The foods you ate most often are the most likely suspects for allergies/intolerances. If when you do this, you think, "I'd really miss that if I had to cut it out," or if you're aware of having a craving for something, then it's even more of a suspect.

Elimination Diet

For a trial period of a month, or until the symptoms have clearly improved, cut out the food that you think may be causing your allergies. Observe what happens to your symptoms, but bear in mind that, just like an addict going "cold turkey," you may feel worse before you feel better. If there's no improvement, and no worsening either, by the end of a month, you haven't identified the trigger or not all of them. You have to be prepared to do this 100 percent, though, because even a tiny amount of a food can set off a reaction. Sometimes, especially when trying to help a child with an allergy, you may need to get the whole family off the food, and even to remove it entirely from your home, so there's no temptation calling from behind the pantry door.

If you do improve, you can confirm the reaction by challenging yourself with a small amount of the food—if the symptoms return, that's your proof. Remember that this may take twenty-four hours or more to happen. *Warning:* be careful, however, if you have any

THE GLUTEN-FREE DIET

A gluten-free diet is not the same as a wheat-free diet. Gluten is most of the protein in wheat, about 80 percent, but it is different from the other proteins because it is bound to the starch, the carbohydrate that is the biggest part of the wheat seed. Making wheat gluten-free is easy: you just wash away the starch and the gluten goes with it. The other proteins are in the living "embryo" part of the seed.

A wheat-free diet is not a gluten-free diet either. There is a small amount of gluten in all the other grains that we use—barley, rye, oats (though this is argued about), and even spelt. To go gluten-free, you need to avoid all of these as well as wheat. Buckwheat is from a different family and is free of gluten.

of the symptoms listed in Chapter 2, because reintroducing the food could be dangerous, so don't do it. Just stay off the food.

CHEMICAL SENSITIVITIES

Chemical sensitivities are more like inhalant allergies than food reactions, in that it is hard to miss what's going on and hard to avoid them too. I don't need to tell you how to spot a reaction to tobacco smoke or to vehicle exhaust, for instance. You already know about it. Diagnosing a problem with chemical fumes probably won't be difficult.

You might want to go back and read the information in Chapter 1 about mold, however. It is a problem that is difficult to classify (is it an allergy or is it a toxicity? an inhalant or a chemical?) and sometimes difficult to find the source.

It may prove difficult to avoid and remove most chemical fumes, but that's where the rest of this book should come in handy. It makes sense to clean out your house and make it a safe haven, as much as you can. If you haven't done this already, go through your home and collect all the chemicals, cleaning fluids, aerosols, perfumes, and solvents, and throw them out. Dispose of them responsibly, of course, and recycle where possible or give them to someone who will use them.

Some people find that wearing a mask helps when out in town, but it usually doesn't help a lot. These days, with swine flu and all the other health scares, masks don't look so weird as they once did. I'll be telling you more about how to deal with chemical sensitivities in later chapters.

MY PERSONAL EXPERIENCE WITH ALLERGIES

I used to be intolerant of milk (see the box "Loss of Insight" in Chapter 1). I gave it up for about three years. Every few months, I had a little bit to check whether I still reacted, and when I didn't I started having little bits of cheese and small amounts of milk. Even today, I don't push it, so I never have cereal with milk, for instance. Of course, all this time I have been using nutritional approaches as best I can, which have helped. I could have used a desensitization technique for milk, but it never seemed worth it.

I did desensitize myself for hay fever. This was a problem when I was at school, then hardly noticeable during medical school (I guess I didn't get out much), but it came back in my thirties. One year, I had a first floor office right next to the park, and it was such a high-pollen summer you could see the stuff drifting along in the sunlight. My symptoms returned, so before the next year's season, I gave myself the desensitization shots and it didn't happen again. Vitamin C and other nutrients helped, and still do, and it's never come back in a big way.

CHAPTER 5

GENES, POLLUTION, AND DIET

Since the Human Genome Project was completed in 2003, we have entered a new era of health care—personalized medicine. The "old" genetics was about telling you, "your baby has Down syndrome" or "you have a 25 percent chance of developing what your father had." It was based on big changes in your genes, or your DNA (deoxyribonucleic acid). The new genomics makes it possible for us to tell you that "your genes give you an increased risk of heart disease or allergies or some other disease, but here's what you can do about it."

It also enables us to predict the drugs that will work better on you, which is why the pharmaceutical industry is so interested. Genomics is all about how your genes interact with your diet, your environment, and your medications. It is based on very small changes in DNA known as SNiPs—single nucleotide polymorphisms. Nucleotides are the letters of DNA, the units that spell out the whole word that tells the cell exactly what molecule to build. You may have seen illustrations of a part of the human genome, which is 3,200,000,000 nucleotides long. If stretched out straight, the human genome would be as tall as a person—about six feet. It's just a long sequence of four nucleotides: adenine, cytosine, guanine, and thymine. A SNiP happens when one of these nucleotide sequences is changed, and even a tiny change can make a huge difference.

Every cell has 23,000 genes in its nucleus, and we only know anything worth knowing about less than 100 of them. But scientists are busy studying as many genes as they can to learn what they tell us about how the body works, how we fall sick, and how to treat it. Nearly all of your genes involve nutrition in some way, because the protein molecules that the genes produce are for dealing with the atoms and molecules that you eat (vitamins, minerals, proteins, and fats), and at the same time these proteins are made from what you eat. One potential concern with genomics research, and the profit-driven businesses that fund it, is that it will be mainly focused on how your genes affect the way that drugs work in the body, and not in how they affect the way nutrients work. Patentable drug-based interventions are likely to be chosen over diet- and lifestyle-based ones, and treatments may be chosen over prevention.

GENOMICS AND ALLERGIES

You're reading this because you've got an allergy, so how does genomics affect you? Well, there are visible effects and hidden effects. The visible one is that you may have inherited the genes for an allergy or for a problem that makes allergy more likely. You can figure this out for yourself simply by doing your family history. Just map out a family tree, and include all the diseases and medical problems that everyone had; ask your parents about their illnesses and their parents' illnesses, and those of your aunts and uncles.

So if your father has hay fever and your mother had eczema as a child, you are much more likely to develop an atopic disease (asthma, eczema, urticaria, hay fever, rhinitis). If you are female, and both your mother and her mother had thyroid disease, then both you and your daughters are more likely to have this problem at some stage in your life. And provided you don't develop any serious gynecological problems, the age at which your mother went through menopause is a good indicator of when you can expect to do so. For men, if your father got heart disease at an early age, you may well be at risk of doing so. Your paternal grandfather may have lived long enough ago that he wasn't exposed to the same dietary and environmental factors as you, so what happened to him is less important than your father and uncles.

Remember, though, that genes are no longer seen as destiny—there is always something you can do about it. Most of the time, both with heart disease and with allergies, as with nearly all health issues, they can be influenced by diet and nutrition, lifestyle, and exercise choices that you make.

The hidden effect of genomics on allergies has to do with the environment and with how your body handles environmental toxins. We all have a number of genes coding for the proteins, called enzymes, that deal with getting rid of the molecules we don't need, both the products of normal metabolism and the toxins that we are all exposed to in our food, water, and air. But these genes vary in ways that can make a big difference, and many of us have such SNiPs. The difference the SNiPs make is in just how efficient you are at inactivating and getting rid of toxins, at detoxifying.

Now, for most of the time that humans have been on earth, this has made no real difference to health. If it had, those with the "bad" SNiPs would have died out, or at least there would be lot fewer of us around. It makes a difference now because the level of toxins we are all exposed to is so much higher, and it's rising all the time. It may be that the children who are developing autism, in increasing numbers of epidemic proportions, are the ones who are less efficient at removing toxic minerals like mercury and lead from their bodies, particularly from their brains. Food intolerances also play a part in autism: at least two-thirds of parents of autistic children who have tried it said that their child got better on a gluten-free, casein-free diet (basically cutting out all wheat and milk).[1]

Your detoxification capacity makes a difference to allergies. In 2006, researchers in California took people who had known pollen allergies, which gave them hay fever, and they exposed them to the pollen and then measured their blood immunoglobulin E (IgE, the major antibody in classic allergies such as hay fever and asthma). On some occasions, they exposed them to second-hand tobacco smoke or to exhaust fumes just before the pollen exposure. One group had polymorphisms (SNiPs) in the *GSTM1* gene, which codes for a major liver detoxification enzyme, while the other group didn't. When exposed to pollen only, they all produced about the same amount of IgE. When exposed to the fumes before the pollen, the subjects with normal *GSTM1* genes, who produced healthy enzymes, made six times as much IgE; however, those with the "null" genes, who didn't produce any functioning enzyme, made fifteen times as much IgE. In other words, environmental pollution will make anybody's allergy worse, but if your body can't detoxify very well, it will make your allergy a lot worse.[2] Another study found that having the same SNiPs greatly increased a child's chances of developing allergic asthma.[3]

So your genetically determined capacity to detoxify makes a big difference to asthma/hay fever types of allergies, both giving you a greater probability of developing the problem in the first place and making it worse when it does happen. It does so because we are all exposed to increasing amounts of chemical pollutants that we need to detoxify. Could this be part of the reason why the number of allergy cases is rising so rapidly?

Detoxification ability has even more to do with chemical sensitivities. A Canadian study in 2004 found that people with a certain combination of two SNiPs were over eighteen times more likely to have multiple chemical sensitivity (MCS), a chronic medical condition caused by low levels of exposure to multiple chemicals.[4] A German study found a similar result, looking at a different set of genes.[5] The enzymes coded for by the affected genes in both studies were detoxification enzymes.

The worse your body is at detoxifying, the more likely you are to develop allergy problems. We now know this to be true for the classic allergies like asthma and hay fever, and it is also true for chemical sensitivities. We can't yet say the same is true of food

A COMPLEX ALLERGY CASE

Chris is a big, athletic 45-year-old lawyer who had a lot of ear and throat "infections" as a child, for which he was given several courses of antibiotics. In his twenties, when he started playing a lot of sports, he developed persistent fatigue, brain fog, and bouts of night sweats. Tests confirmed his suspicion of food intolerances. He was treated successfully with nutrition and a course of desensitization, and he stayed well for several years (provided that he didn't overdo things). Then he had a sudden relapse after exposure to, and becoming sensitized to, the chemicals in a newly decorated office. A single experiment with marijuana caused him to become acutely allergic to that as well. He was able to take a year off from work and remained relatively well during this time, traveling and relaxing. On returning to work, though, he struggled with low-grade symptoms and fatigue.

In the last three years, investigations have shown Chris to have:

- Intestinal parasites and a leaky gut (treating these improved his health, but not a lot)

- Increased levels of pesticides and flame retardants in his fat cells

- Genomic changes (SNiPs) in his liver detoxification enzymes

Thus, a number of factors conspired to make him unwell, and he has had to take an integrated approach to getting well again. Chris is now in the process of removing toxins from his system, slowly but surely, and he still gets regular desensitizing shots. He continues to minimize his exposure to his known allergens, and he eats a healthy diet and takes nutritional supplements.

His genomic testing results enabled him to make some adjustments to diet and lifestyle, with some unexpected benefits. For example, some vegetables are good for him, some are clearly bad for him, for genetic reasons not allergic ones. It is now a question of using all the information he has—on his genes, his pollutant exposures, his nutrition, and his allergies—to manage his health for the long-term.

intolerances, because the research hasn't been done yet, but a link may potentially be found.

WHAT CAN YOU DO?

Knowing what we do so far, it's clear there are two simple, basic ways of tackling your built-in tendency to allergies:

- Minimize your exposure to chemicals

- Optimize your nutritional status

Minimize Your Exposure to Chemicals

Chemicals are harmful to health not just if you're allergic to them, but because they can also clog up your system, overload your detoxification pathways, and make all kinds of allergies worse. Exposure to chemicals is also a factor in a number of chronic illnesses and probably increases your risk of being overweight or getting heart disease and cancer.

Completely avoiding chemicals just isn't possible. In fact, some chemically sensitive people find it difficult to have a regular life because they try to live in a chemical-free bubble. The problem with that strategy is the same one that astronauts have—re-entry. Coming back to earth, to real life, can be painful and even dangerous, because all the body systems that have been able to take a rest (the muscles that have been free of gravity or the enzymes free of chemicals) have to be forced, protesting, back to work. I don't mean that it is always wrong to lock yourself away from the world, but it should probably be the last resort. Also, if you stay the course in the real world, you may help make things a bit easier for those who come after you, of whom there will be many.

So, practically speaking, you can't completely avoid chemicals, but you can minimize your exposure to them. You can clean up your diet, your water, and your indoor environment.

Clean Up Your Diet

There have recently been news stories about organic food. The U.K.'s Food Standards Agency released a review of the scientific evidence on organic foods claiming that they have no more of the important nutrients than ordinary foods. Of course, what the headlines screamed was "Organic No Better for Health." Now, I've been buying organic foods for years, where and when I can, not for the increased vitamins but for the absence of toxic, polluting chemicals such as pesticides. And not only because it's good for my health, but because it's good for the planet too.

Michael Pollan, author of *In Defense of Food: An Eater's Manifesto,* advised not to eat anything unpronounceable. He put it another way too—don't eat anything your great-grandmother wouldn't recognize as food—that is, avoiding all the chemicals that industrialized food production has introduced into the food chain. The same goes for beverages. Cleaning up your diet can be as simple as that.

Simple doesn't always mean easy, however. When your body has been fooled by synthetic ingredients and too much sugar in foods for a long time, your palate may need some retraining. You need to allow time to adjust to the taste of real food again. One trick that may help is to set up your own tasting sessions: try a natural food and the processed equivalent side-by-side. But remember always to try the natural one first, because the chemicals in the processed version can deaden your taste buds.

The guidelines for cleaning up your diet are as follows:

- Always read labels and avoid the unpronounceable ingredients.

- Avoid processed foods, because you can't trust them as you would something you prepared yourself. Factory-made food has to have artificial ingredients to make it flow, to stick together, and so on.

- Eat and drink organic as much as you can, although a good local producer who you know and trust can be just as good and

.cheaper. Organic foods help you (and the planet) reduce your exposure to toxic chemicals.

• Support your local health food store and farmers' market, rather than the supermarket.

Clean Up Your Water

You need a daily intake of good, clean water to help your body flush out toxins, the by-products of digestion, and the breakdown products of recycling and repair in your cells. If you are going to be somewhere hot or doing something hot in the sun, you will lose water through perspiration and breathing, and you need to replace this as well.

Unfortunately, tap water may not be the best source, and you can't believe everything the water utilities tell you. They often say that their tap water is as pure as is possible. What they mean is that the water is bacteriologically pure—there aren't any bugs in it—which is true, but it's only part of the truth. The water from your tap is probably loaded with chemicals (necessary to kill the bugs) that alter the taste and may even be harmful for your health. Most of this toxicity originates from the chlorine that is added to sterilize the water. Chlorine then interacts with chemicals that are added to, or even that occur naturally in, the water to form toxic substances. Of course, in many places, chemicals from industrial pollution or from agricultural run-off end up in the mix, making something even more toxic.

The good news is that proper water filters, based on activated charcoal or on reverse osmosis, are reasonably good at removing most of the pollutants in water, including the chlorine compounds. It is worthwhile having a filter installed at home—a plumbed-in one is best, but jug filters can still be useful provided you follow the instructions. If you use them a lot, though, jug-based water filters are hard work and more expensive in the end. Use the water for all cooking purposes, as well as for drinking and making tea, coffee, and other beverages.

The purest water you can get is good mineral water. Whereas the best you can do with tap water is to clean it up again, mineral waters should have been in the ground for so long that they are effectively preindustrial, and in any case they have been filtered through several hundred feet of solid rock, the biggest and best filter in the world. They may also have the advantage of containing extra minerals, such as calcium and magnesium. While you may select your mineral water with mineral supplementation in mind, its main value is purity and lack of toxins, so you can use it to wash your inside every day just as you do your outside. However, consider the transportation miles and energy costs involved in getting it to you—choose one that's indigenous and preferably that comes from your own state. (Check the website www.mineral waters.org, which catalogues over 3,000 different mineral waters from around the world.[6])

Opinions vary on how much water you should drink, and to be honest, nobody knows for certain. My advice is to not trust anybody who claims to have all the answers. Alternative practitioners can sometimes be just as patronizing as ordinary doctors. From experience, I would suggest that adults aim to drink at least 1 liter (about a quart) of pure water daily.

The guidelines for cleaning up your water are:

- Get and use a water filtration system or filter pitcher for the tap water you use in cooking and for drinking.

- Drink mineral water as well.

Clean Up Your Indoor Environment

There is a theory about allergies called the "hygiene hypothesis," which can be summarized as follows:

- Exposure to lots of infectious agents in childhood is healthy for kids' immune systems; it's what they were designed for.

- We have all cleaned up our homes too much, and we should let our kids eat a bit of dirt now and then.

- Their immune systems would develop a bit of strength, be better at resisting infections, and so wouldn't bother inventing unnecessary allergic reactions.

Nobody has really tested this theory, and there is one big problem with it—dirt just isn't what it used to be. When I was at

ECOLOGICAL MEDICINE

If you're wondering what kind of doctor I am, I'm not a mainstream allergist—what I practice is known as ecological medicine. It is scientific medicine that looks at how individual humans interact with the environment. We can identify several components of this, and the thing that strikes me as I write this is just how much they have all changed, both the facts and our understanding of them, in the time I have been practicing medicine.

Allergy—Alterations in the way our immune systems handle outside factors that are hard to avoid, such as foods, chemicals, and pollens.

Nutrition—The supply, good or bad, of those things we have to take in to survive, including vitamins, minerals, essential fats, and so on.

Toxicity—Things that we mine or manufacture that end up in water and food, and so in our bloodstreams and inside our cells, which can interfere with functioning.

Biochemical Individuality—We're learning quickly about the genomic part of this, which has a large effect on allergy and toxicity, and so on our health.

Ecology and Sustainability—Spending on health in the United States runs at 16 percent of gross domestic product (that's one dollar in every six). What does that tell us about its carbon footprint and pollution footprint? We each have a responsibility for the planet.

medical school long ago, we were taught that indoor dirt was made up in large part of human skin debris, plus stray food, bits of soft furnishings, and so on. That's no longer true. We tend to think of dirt as dusty, dry stuff, but the dirt inside our homes has a large enough oil component that it forms an oily film on any surface. It's made up of oils from us, from cooking, and from exhaust pollution. Because most of the environmental pollutants around us are fat-soluble (that's why the first step in the body's detoxification and excretion process is to make them water-soluble), they will absorb into that film. Every time someone touches the surface, they pick up a bit of both the oil and the pollutants, and they are easily absorbed into the bloodstream.

Some recent studies looked at the levels of PBDEs (polybrominated diphenyl ethers), or flame retardants that must be put in soft furnishings by law; some of the boards in your computer may be as much as 40 percent flame retardant. The researchers found levels of PBDEs that were 20 times higher inside houses than outside.[7] Inside airplanes, they found high levels as well. Human blood levels corresponded to the levels inside their houses, but children had around ten times the blood levels of adults. That's because they crawl around and put their hands in their mouths a lot. And the enzymes that detoxify these chemicals are nowhere near as efficient in kids as adults: overall, down to a quarter or a third of the activity per unit of blood in babies, but in the kids whose genes had SNiPs, the enzymes were even lower.[8]

So, this tells us that "feeding your child a bit of dirt" is no longer an option, but also, more worryingly, that they are already taking in significant amounts of toxins that way. As are we all. There's nobody on this planet, apart from a few tribespeople up the Amazon, whose body isn't still carrying around some of the pesticide DDT (dichlorodiphenyltrichloroethane) and its metabolites,[9] even though it is banned in most places (in the U.S. since 1972) apart from its use in malaria prevention. No wonder it is called a persistent organic pollutant.

If you want to do the best you can at avoiding chemicals, follow these suggestions:

- Empty your kitchen cupboard of all chemical-based cleaning fluids and replace them with eco-friendly products. But remember that green doesn't always mean chemical-free, or vice versa.

- Empty your bathroom cabinet of all chemical-based cosmetics and toiletries and find more natural alternatives.

- Educate your hairdresser or beauty parlor if they don't know about chemical-free, scent-free hair colorants, treatments, skin cleansers, and so on. You probably won't be the first person to raise the issue with them.

- Be careful with new furnishings and drapes—they are required by law to contain flame retardants. It is best to use old ones, if possible; failing that, leave new items opened out in the garage or somewhere for a couple of weeks to "outgas."

- Be very careful with new carpets and flooring as they are likely to contain adhesives and solvents that can be toxic. Minimize these, if possible, and after installation leave the room unoccupied for a couple of weeks with good ventilation and intermittent heating.

- Likewise, new computers, printers, and copiers should be left switched on, to run them hot, for at least a few days to outgas.

Optimize Your Nutritional Status

In the next chapter, we'll look at using nutritional supplements for fighting allergies, but here are some basics about improving your diet. Most of this is the same as the instructions for avoiding chemicals in food, but there's one big addition about carbohydrates.

Eat Traditionally Grown Foods

If you buy your food from a farmers' market instead of from a supermarket, in addition to containing fewer chemicals, it will likely be fresher because it hasn't traveled hundreds (or thousands) of miles to get to you. The vitamins and oils in the food will have had less time to break down, so you will be getting more of these nutrients in every mouthful. Also, a lot of supermarket foods are now grown hydroponically (in water with added nutrients) and have never touched soil. You are a more complex organism than a cucumber, and there are some nutrients you need that the cucumber doesn't, but there's no reason for the growers to put them in either the soil or the hydroponic mix.

Analyzing the nutrient content of foods is a tricky business, and comparing organic to conventional foods much more so. For a start, farmers learn and change their techniques all the time, and conventional farmers often learn tricks from organic farmers. So it's not surprising that you can find research that favors both sides. The best review I have found was done by The Organic Center, established by the Organic Trade Association, based in Greenfield, Massachusetts. The report, available online, is rigorous and impressive and looked at levels of nine key nutrients in 187 foods.[10]

- Two-thirds of the comparisons found that organic foods had more nutrients.

- One-third found that conventional food had more.

- Averaging them all out, organic food had 25 percent more nutrients than conventional.

I encourage you to buy "traditionally grown" food rather than organic, though. Traditionally grown means that a farmer, who you can probably speak to at a farmers' market, knows all about the food. He or she may even know the names of the animals and grew or raised the food with respect for nature and for the animals, and with a low ecological impact. And if it isn't certified organic it will still probably be close to it.

Cook Your Own Food

When you buy fresh food and cook it yourself, the field-to-plate time is shorter than for a processed or prepared food, and you can also cook it in ways that don't break down the nutrients or flush them out of the food. Steaming vegetables is the best way to keep their nutritional value. Don't microwave them, though, as this does break down some of the enzymes and proteins in food. Using a microwave oven is fine for heating up a cup of tea, but not for real food.

Reduce Your Intake of Sugar and Carbohydrates

I like a coffee in the morning—just one, you understand. I was in line at the coffee shop recently, behind a large lady who asked for "a decaf skinny latte with two sugars please." So that's take out the caffeine, take out the fats, and put in extra sugar! That's what's wrong with our diet in a nutshell. I see patients all the time who have deficiencies of essential fats in their bodies, but I've never seen one with a deficiency of sugar. (Okay, I've seen some anorexics, but they are deficient in everything.)

For way too long, the food industry has been selling us the line that all fat is bad, and then selling us the "solution." They're wrong. Fats (lipids) are essential to life. Yes, they contain calories, but they are also vital building blocks for every cell in our bodies. Every cell has a cell wall that keeps some substances in and others out, and lets them in and out when necessary. These walls are made up of oils. And even cholesterol is an important component oil. Get too little of these oils and your body gets sick.

At the same time, we have been sold the line that sugar is essential for energy. That's wrong too. Primarily our bodies are designed to use oils for energy in the tiny structures called mitochondria that are inside every cell. This is also part of the "housekeeping" in cells, which breaks down and burns the damaged or undesirable fats. We also have the mechanisms for using sugars (such as insulin from the pancreas), but they are meant to be a back-up, switched on when necessary, not to work flat-out the whole time, which is what happens when you eat too many sugars.

Diabetes happens when your body doesn't handle sugar properly. But diabetes is really two very different diseases, known as type I and type II. Type I diabetes, which usually happens early in life, is an autoimmune disease in which the body develops an "allergy" to its own tissues—in this case, to cells in the pancreas. It makes up less than 10 percent of diabetes cases. Type II diabetes is due to insulin resistance, and it is probably better described as the "metabolic syndrome." Forty-seven million Americans suffer from metabolic syndrome. And it comes from eating and drinking too much sugar. To be diagnosed with the metabolic syndrome, you need to have central obesity, high blood sugar, and signs of cardiovascular disease (high blood pressure, high cholesterol, and the like).

All of these problems are linked, of course, and they are clearly linked to too many calories and/or too little exercise. The excess calories in our diet come mainly from sugar and carbohydrates. When you eat too many of these, the body first stores them in fat cells next to the intestine. That's why the obesity occurs mainly around the waist. When this area becomes full, the body starts storing fat in the liver and then everywhere else. It's insulin that pushes sugar into cells, but when they start getting full the insulin doesn't work any more—this is called insulin resistance. Insulin also pushes other, more essential, nutrients into the cell: amino acids, vitamin C, and magnesium, in particular. So, when a cell is insulin resistant, it gets starved of these nutrients as well.

It would be remarkable if all this didn't affect the immune system. It does: a dose of sugar effectively stuns the white blood cells, making them less effective at tackling infections. Sugar also messes up the normal flora in the bowel—the billions of "friendly" bacteria in the intestines that are necessary to health—and can make the bowel more leaky, so food allergens get across and irritate the immune system. And sugar causes a stress response in the body, which can trigger the immune system and lead to allergies.

Genuine allergies to sugar probably do happen, but they are uncommon compared to reactions to wheat, milk, corn, and the other major ones. There are so many other reasons why too much sugar is a bad idea—worry about them first!

To summarize, in order to optimize your nutritional status, you should:

- Buy traditionally grown foods, not industrial foods.

- Buy local and meet the farmer.

- Cook your own food to preserve the nutrients.

- Eat meals—don't graze.

- Cut out added sugar, especially sugary soft drinks.

- Cut down on refined carbohydrates; eat whole grains instead.

CHAPTER 6

NUTRITION FOR ALLERGIES

We've talked about preventing allergies, but you can't always do that. What if it's ragweed pollen that's making you sneeze, for instance? Moving out of the city, away from the pollution, would seem a good idea, but it might just expose you to more pollen, making you worse off. Or what if you have a chemical sensitivity, but you can't avoid the chemicals completely and still live in your city and go to your job? In this chapter, we're going to look at supplements you can take to reduce or even switch off the symptoms you get when exposed to your allergens. I'll also give you guidelines about how much of each to take and how often.

The simplest way to use this advice is to take all of the nutrients, and this will certainly help most people. But this isn't always necessary or practical.

- You may not need all of the supplements all of the time. And they don't come for free, of course. If cost is an issue, or if being able to take something several times a day is tricky, you are free to experiment and see what you can get away with. It's your body and your symptoms after all. Important exceptions to this are when it's a serious reaction—never take chances with those (see Chapter 2: Allergies That Kill).

- Conversely, you may need more of some of them. The worse the allergy, the more you need, in general. It takes lots more vitamin C to make an impact on asthma, for instance, than it does on hay fever. Body weight is also a consideration a 200-pound person is bound to need around twice as much of a nutrient as a 100-pound person. Finally, where are you starting from? How bad is your nutrition and health to begin with? The worse it is, the more of these vitamins and supplements you're likely to need to reach the ideal level. And if you have other health problems going on at the same time, it's likely to take longer to correct your deficiencies.

So, I'm never going to be able to tell you *exactly* what will work for you, only approximately. You'll always need to do some tweaking, some fine-tuning. Which is a good thing, because doing that will give you three things:

- A better awareness of what is going on in your own body—These days, we spend so much time looking at and thinking about the road ahead, the computer screen, and the world we live in that it's easy to lose touch with the world inside us. But every symptom means something, and it's good to learn again to spot the signs and read them.

- An understanding of how all these factors interact on your body —Do you need the supplements more when you can't maintain a good diet, for instance? Or when you're under stress? Some runners found that they hit a wall of abdominal cramps after a few miles, but if they cut wheat out of their diet, it just didn't happen.

- A better sense of control over your health—Wouldn't it be good to know that when an allergy problem happens you can deal with it yourself, rather than being dependent on a doctor? Better to be master of your own health than to have to get checked in for servicing like a car, to have someone looking under the hood all the time and trying to fix things.

NUTRIENTS ALL WORK TOGETHER

When you take anything to stop a disease or a symptom of a disease, you're working on a chain reaction, a series of interconnected biochemical events that end up producing an effect in your body. If what you're taking is a drug, you're usually aiming to block the effect, and you only have to block one step in the chain reaction to do that. But with nutrition, you're usually trying to get the entire chain of reactions working properly again, and that often means having to get each step working, which may require a whole list of nutrients. It's a more complex thing you're trying to do, but it's more natural too.

This means that giving a lot of just one nutrient may not work, so you have to call for back-up. Whenever you take any of the vitamins, minerals, and other nutrients recommended in this book, it makes sense to have your insurance policy in place by taking a good multivitamin/multimineral as well.

Some nutrients stay in the body for weeks and months, while others are gone in hours. Most of the slow-burners are fat-soluble, and the fast-burners are water-soluble. For instance, when taking omega-3 essential fatty acids, you may need to wait three months before you see an effect. The flip-side is that a single, large dose of vitamin A or vitamin D will work for three months. Vitamin C is in the water-soluble, fast-burner group, and you need to take it several times per day to keep it working.

SIDE EFFECTS

I've been working with allergies and nutrition for nearly thirty years now and I think I've got a pretty good understanding of the risks of supplementation. Yes, there are risks, and if somebody ever tells you that what they're doing is *completely* safe and risk-free, my advice is to stay away from them. If something can be used for good, it can usually do harm as well.

I've spent a lot of time in recent years, together with colleagues, examining and criticizing a lot of reports of adverse effects from nutritional supplements and proposed regulations to limit the doses you are allowed to take. Most of it is rubbish science:

the numbers are distorted in the scientific paper, then a journal hype it a bit more, and then the media hype it a whole lot more, screaming "Vitamins kill!" Don't believe everything you read.

In this book, where there is a possible side effect of anything I'm recommending, I will tell you. It will be a minor side effect, because if there was a serious one I would not be recommending that supplement.

CAUTION: STEARATES

There is a minor but tiresome side effect that you should know about—a small number of allergy sufferers show a reaction to the additive chemicals in many supplement tablets and capsules. This is fairly common, and it's a good reason to find the purest supplements you can. Perhaps the most common additive for people to react to are stearates, usually magnesium stearate or calcium stearate. They are used as lubricants in the manufacture of a lot of tablets and capsules (pharmaceuticals as well as supplements) because they help powders to flow through the encapsulating machines. That's why manufacturers are reluctant to ditch them, even though they can cause problems. A few do manage it, but of course you will pay more for stearate-free supplements.

I don't know whether stearates can cause real allergies, and I doubt that at tiny doses in supplements they are toxic.[1] However, if you find yourself taking more than, say, ten different supplements every day, you should remember that what you are taking most of is the additives like stearates that are in all or most of them, and they could have an effect on your biochemistry over a period of weeks. Some people get symptoms from them at small doses too; if this happens to you, you'll need to avoid them and all the other chemicals that are put into capsules and tablets.

VITAMIN C

Ascorbic acid (ascorbate or vitamin C) is essential to life. But humans are unusual: unlike most animals and organisms, we can't make our own, so we have to get it from food. If we get seriously deficient in it, we develop the disease known as scurvy.

In 1747, a ship's surgeon in the British Royal Navy, James Lind, conducted what is reckoned to be the first controlled scientific trial—he gave oranges and lemons every day to some of the sailors on his ship and not to the rest, and he showed conclusively that this prevented them from developing scurvy. It took another forty-eight years before his findings were accepted and acted on by the navy. They eventually used limes, which were more readily available, for this purpose; hence, the reason Brits are sometimes referred to as "limeys." British explorer Captain James Cook (1728–1779), on his voyages that "discovered" Hawaii, achieved the same effect with sauerkraut (fermented cabbage). You don't get much vitamin C in fermented cabbage or in an orange that's been in a barrel for weeks, but you don't need much to prevent scurvy. Untreated, however, it will kill you through a combination of uncontrolled bleeding and lack of resistance to infection.

Preventing scurvy is not the only thing that vitamin C can do for you, but you need a lot of ascorbic acid to get all the benefits. Here are some of the benefits of vitamin C:

- Fighting infections—White blood cells use a lot of vitamin C when they are activated to tackle infections, and it works. Used correctly, vitamin C will reduce the severity and duration of the symptoms of the common cold.[2] It even works well for viruses like swine flu and for pneumonia and other complications that can occur.[3]

- Fighting cancer—It is clear that having a decent level of vitamin C in your diet can greatly reduce your risk of developing cancer.[4] The trail-blazing studies by Nobel Prize–winner Linus Pauling, Ph.D., and Ewan Cameron, M.D., in the 1970s showed that high doses could also treat, or at least slow down, cancer.[5] Despite many attempts to discredit it, and the shameful lack of a controlled trial, these results have been confirmed, not least by orthomolecular physician Abram Hoffer, M.D., Ph.D.[6]

- Fighting heart disease—Having more vitamin C in your diet and your system can reduce your risk of dying from cardiovascular problems by about 40 percent.[7]

- Strengthening tissues—Vitamin C is necessary for making collagen, which is in the connective tissue that holds your body together. Without enough ascorbate, you will be much more prone to back problems, arthritis, and even physical aging.

- Improving mineral absorption—Some iron tablets for anemia have vitamin C in them, as absorption of iron, magnesium, and other minerals is helped by it.

- Blocking toxins—High intakes of vitamin C protect against the damage caused by most toxins, including heavy metals like lead and mercury, as well as petrochemicals, pesticides, and so on. Ascorbic acid helps you to flush toxins out of the body, and it blocks the toxic effects in a number of ways.

- Protects from shock—Very large doses of vitamin C can prevent anaphylaxis and other kinds of dangerous reactions from developing.[8]

- Antioxidant—Vitamin C protects the water-based parts of your body from free radicals.

- Anti-inflammatory and anti-allergic—When the body detects damage, it sends both histamine and vitamin C to the site. The first opens up the blood vessels and produces inflammation (necessary for healing); ascorbate moderates the potentially dangerous effects of histamine and at the same time protects tissues from free radical damage.[9]

It's the last two effects that we are primarily interested in here—stopping inflammation and stopping allergies. Histamine is the main chemical the body uses to produce allergy symptoms, and vitamin C is its safeguard, the main antihistamine chemical. Since the body uses it naturally, you can surely use it to control your allergies too.

Dose

The pioneering researchers on vitamin C found out early on that the dose was critical. For instance, 100 mg of vitamin C did little or nothing for hay fever, 500 mg was variable in effect but worked for most patients,[10] but 2,000 mg or more was even better.[11] Now, a lot of research that has been used to demonstrate that ascorbic acid doesn't work has used (deliberately?) too small a dose. That's how many sought to discredit the work of Dr. Pauling, who was the first to spread the word about large doses of vitamin C to the world.

Animals that produce their own vitamin C, unlike humans, produce a lot, the equivalent of tens of grams in a human. When you are unwell, you need more vitamin C as fuel for your white blood cells, as antioxidant protection, and for many other reasons. So you tolerate more ascorbic acid. I've experimented on myself and discovered the following:

I weigh approximately 195 pounds (89 kilograms). When I'm well, I can handle 6 grams of vitamin C per day. When getting a cold, this increases to around 12 grams. With the flu, I can get through 20–25 grams without a problem. I've personally not been sicker than that for a long time, but I have heard of severely ill people tolerating 200 grams of vitamin C a day and keeping the illness at bay with it.

This fits with what some of the early researchers determined about ascorbic acid dosing. Frederick Klenner, MD, wrote a number of papers about vitamin C from the 1940s through to the early

1970s. He reported that mild infections could be dealt with by using 65 mg of vitamin C per kilogram of body weight, more severe ones might need 250 mg/kg, and doses much higher than this were safe. We regularly give 75 grams of vitamin C intravenously, without problems so far.

TITRATING VITAMIN C TO BOWEL TOLERANCE

Titrating to bowel tolerance is a way to achieve the maximum intake of ascorbic acid without side effects like diarrhea.

First, dissolve 2 grams (half a level teaspoonful) of vitamin C powder (ascorbic acid or buffered ascorbate) in 2 fluid ounces of water or juice. Drink the liquid. Repeat this every 30 minutes until watery bowel motions occur (as if you had taken an enema). If watery bowel motions have not occurred after a full day of this, begin again in the morning, this time at one level teaspoonful (4 g) in 2 ounces of water or juice every 15 minutes. When watery bowel motions occur, stop consuming the ascorbate for that day.

Next, calculate the total ascorbate consumed during the day. For example, 2 g x 12 doses = 24 g. Or 4 g x 22 doses = 88 g. Whatever your total dose, around three-quarters of this level is your approximate daily need (bowel tolerance). Consume this as liquid, tablets, or capsules, in four or more doses per day. The aim is to achieve a consistent level of vitamin C in your bloodstream.

As you get healthier, the useful life span of ascorbate inside your body will increase, and less will be needed to achieve the desired effect. Then you can reduce your intake; indeed, you will need to, as less is needed to produce watery bowel motions.

Dissolving vitamin C in a larger quantity of liquid may be easier than making up a small batch every time. Use a sealable bottle, such as a mineral water bottle. Dissolved ascorbate is stable for a day but no longer, if it is kept in a sealed bottle, under refrigeration when possible.

There's nothing that says you have to figure the dose by titrating to bowel tolerance (see box), but it does let you know how much is enough and how much is too much. If you don't want to follow that route and you have an allergy or other symptom that you need to control, then use that as your marker instead—when the symptom goes away, or at least gets easier to tolerate, then that's about the level you need.

If you're self-administering vitamin C, it will have to be by mouth. In the past, people used intramuscular injections, but they are painful so you need a local anesthetic with the vitamin; I don't know anybody who does them these days. Taking C intravenously is a good way to get a large dose, but this needs to be done in a clinic. (Apparently in Japan you can buy tights impregnated with vitamin C: good for the skin, they say, but not of much use for allergies.)

The oral route for vitamin C is currently being revolutionized by the arrival of liposomal forms. A liposome is an extremely small globule of oil, and if you put a tiny dose of vitamin C inside each globule, they get absorbed quickly and easily, not only from the gut but almost certainly through the skin. I haven't seen proof that the skin route works, but I can't see why it wouldn't.

If you take ordinary water-soluble vitamin C and a liposomal version, they are absorbed into the bloodstream by different routes, so you get more by using two parallel channels. Some doctors and researchers have done the experiment on themselves, and it works.[12] We have yet to figure out what's the best combination and so on, so I'll have to wing this a bit. Another consideration is that the liposomal form is expensive. Up to 16 grams a day (that's a level teaspoon every 6 hours) should be fine with ordinary vitamin C powder.

Side Effects

The only potentially serious side effect that taking a lot of vitamin C *may* do is to increase your risk of kidney stones. About

10–15 percent of us will get a kidney stone at some time in our lives, and one study found that people with high intakes of vitamin C appeared to increase their risk of developing stones.[13] But there are a lot of other factors that make you more likely to get a stone; dehydration is the most obvious. Taking too little magnesium was just as bad as taking too much C; too little potassium was even worse. These are all common dietary deficiencies and another example of nutrients all working together. However, two other large studies found no such effect from vitamin C,[14] so my advice is to make sure you get enough magnesium and potassium and all the other nutrients, whether you're taking lots of vitamin C or not.

A much more common side effect is diarrhea or loose bowels. This is often used by regulators to try to ban vitamin C intakes above around 2,000 mg per day. But actually this is something you can take advantage of—if you get loose bowels, this tells you that you're taking more than the maximum vitamin C your body can use. So you can notch it down until the side effect disappears, and that is your optimum dose. See the box on the previous page "Titrating Vitamin C to Bowel Tolerance" for how to do this.

Guidelines

- Don't underestimate the dose; if most animals were your body weight, they would be generating their own vitamin C at a rate of 10 to 20 grams on a good day (much more on a bad one).

- Take C several times a day at least; the blood level peaks around two hours after swallowing, after which it's down all the way.

- Never put it in boiling water, because this inactivates the vitamin immediately.

- If you need more than around 16 grams per day, use liposomal vitamin C as well.

- If you get loose bowels, you're taking a bit too much.

VITAMIN D

All life comes from the sun. There are factors that we get from the sun indirectly, like food, and factors that we get directly from the sun, like vitamin D, which is formed when ultraviolet (UV) light hits the skin. So what *is* vitamin D? It's called a vitamin, but that's something that we normally have to get from food, not from sunlight. It looks like a hormone, but those are made by our endocrine glands, mainly the adrenals and the ovaries or testes. Vitamin D is a complex, fascinating molecule that affects everything that goes on in our bodies.

Among the functions of vitamin D are the following:

- Makes your muscles stronger, whether you're young or old, fit or frail. In the elderly, it reduces the risk of falls, which can injure and even cause bone fractures.[15]

- Reduces chronic pain—not just low back pain but most, maybe even all, kinds of pain[16]

- Helps to prevent most forms of cancer from developing and may help to slow their progression when they do occur[17]

- Boosts your resistance to infections, including the swine flu and other health panics that occur so often nowadays[18]

- Lifts mood and helps treat depression, including seasonal affective disorder (SAD)[19]

- Strengthens the heart, lowers blood pressure,[20] and reduces the risk of a stroke[21]

- Reduces and delays autoimmune diseases such as multiple sclerosis (MS) and rheumatoid arthritis

Vitamin D and Allergies

Studies involving vitamin D have been mixed, complicated by the fact that researchers often seem to give the wrong dose or measure the wrong molecule. Plus, it can take years for an effect to show. There have been some odd findings; for instance, a Swedish study found that giving children vitamins A and D in a water base doubled their risk of allergies, but the oil-based equivalent had no such effect.[22] Another study found that children who had vitamin D supplements in the first year of life were 50 percent more likely to be allergic at age 31.[23]

One explanation for this could be that they were using the wrong form of vitamin D—vitamin D2 (ergocalciferol), which is not a natural molecule for human bodies (only for yeast organisms) and is nowhere near as potent as vitamin D3, the natural human form. D2 may even block or interfere with vitamin D3. Another insight comes from a British study, which found that both too much and too little vitamin D increased the risk of allergies.[24]

In regard to allergies, we do know that vitamin D:

- Seems to reduce the risk of the most severe anaphylactic reactions[25]

- Reduces the severity of asthma[26]

- Alleviates dermatitis and eczema[27]

- Reduces the risk of autoimmune diseases[28]

- Helps the healing and repair of tissues[29]

We don't know what vitamin D can do directly for food intolerances or chemical sensitivities; nobody has looked at this scientifically. But vitamin D does help to reduce inflammation and repair tissues, especially in mucosal tissue lining the bowel and respiratory tract.

Recent research suggests that you may get a benefit from a combination of vitamins D and C that you don't get from either of them alone.[30] The scientists looked at the free radical damage that occurs when the blood supply to a vital organ is cut off and then released again; this is what happens when you get thrombolytic therapy for your heart attack, for instance. But free radical damage (oxidative stress) is part of every type of inflammation, including allergies. The combination of vitamins C and D improved all the markers in this study. Considering how important free radical damage is as a factor in allergies, combining C and D definitely looks like the way to go.

In my view, everybody needs vitamin D and hardly anybody gets enough, so we should go get it. From sunlight, if you can; if not, take supplements.

Dose

If you read the label on most vitamin pills or on fortified milk or other foods, you'll see that they nearly all consider that around 400 IU (international units) of vitamin D per day is all you need. That was the standard scientific view until a few years ago. Then,

---

CAN YOU GET ENOUGH VITAMIN D FROM SUNSHINE?

Getting enough sunshine to maintain levels of vitamin D depends mainly on where you live. The further north you live, away from the equator, the less ultraviolet (UV) light there is getting through the upper atmosphere—and still less on account of the weather and pollution. When you compare people living in the Northeastern states to the Southwestern states, they get around twice as much cancer, twice as much dental decay, and three times the number of severe allergies.[31]

If you don't live somewhere sunny, it is difficult to get sufficient sunlight to produce enough vitamin D. Even if you do, modern lifestyles mean that most of us only see the sun as we go from our home to our car, or the subway to our office. So, if you live somewhere but don't play a sport or take part in some activity (gardening, walking the dog) that gets you out in the sun with some skin exposed, you may still come up short.

In that case, take vitamin D in supplement form.

several scientists figured out that if you lived like humans did in the Stone Age—in a hot sunny place, outdoors most of the day, without many clothes—you would be manufacturing a lot more than that in your skin every day. More like 10,000 to 20,000 IU a day. And there are benefits to be had from that amount of D which you don't get at lower levels.

For instance, in a study about boosting resistance to infections, taking 800 IU a day reduced the rate of catching influenza and viral infections by 90 percent, but taking 2,000 IU reduced the rate by 97 percent.[32] The point is, take enough—and that means for an adult around 4,000 IU daily. If you weigh over 200 pounds, you should take even higher doses. If you have dark skin and live in a dark place—you're black and live in Chicago, for example—then your risk is even greater, and you should make sure to take this amount even if you don't have allergies.

Some doctors get very worried about overdosing on vitamin D, but the truth is that it never happens. There are no known cases of people dying of an acute overdose of vitamin D (you couldn't really swallow enough pills). Chronic overdose is possible, but you would need to take at least 20,000 IU per day for months on end, so that is pretty rare too. The amount of D you get from sunlight your body naturally regulates, so after the useful point, when you've got around 20,000 IU in a day, more sunlight doesn't raise your vitamin D level. Really, don't worry about ODing; lack of vitamin D, on the other hand, is almost the rule.

Guidelines

- Take about 4,000 IU of vitamin D per day for an adult (half that dose for a child under ten years old, a quarter of that dose for an infant).

- Never take vitamin D2, the ergocalciferol form.

- If you have a day of good sun exposure, you can skip the vitamin D supplement.

- Don't worry about being exactly regular with supplementation; D is a long-acting and slow-acting substance. Missed a day? So what. Missed a week? Take a handful.

- If you're still not sure, get your vitamin D level checked. Your blood level should be at least 40 ng/ml or 100 nmol/L. If it isn't, increase your intake.

ESSENTIAL FATTY ACIDS

It's hard to believe that people are still going on about low-fat diets—and, what's worse, going *on* them—lowering their cholesterol, and taking statins ($30 billion yearly sales worldwide), but they are. It's over thirty years now since the cholesterol hypothesis of heart disease was described, by Professor George Mann in the *New England Journal of Medicine,* as "the greatest scam in the history of medicine."[33] Still, we get low-fat products pushed at us all the time.

Let's get one thing clear—life depends on lipids (fats and oils), *including* cholesterol. Without them, we wouldn't be here. Not just because we burn them to extract the calories, although we do, but because we were designed to run on oil, with sugar and starch just being fuel for the back-up generator. No, more importantly, every cell in your body depends on oils to make the wall surrounding it; and without that wall, it wouldn't be a cell. The cell's wall is what gives it an identity separate from everything else outside. I can't think of a better word than *miraculous* for the composition and function of cell walls. They are functioning the whole time, letting precisely selected molecules in or out, transmitting signals into the cell and onwards to other cells, and maintaining and repairing themselves. So you can imagine that they need a good supply of oils (yes, amino acids, sugars, and other things as well, but mainly oils) to carry on functioning.

You've probably heard a lot lately about the links between inflammation and obesity. It probably also mentioned things like insulin resistance, stress, adrenaline resistance, and leptins. It's simple really: just remember that "excess fat is almost always a sign of inflammation somewhere nearby."[34] Why? Because when your body activates inflammation, it leads to production of either white blood cells, for an immune response, or tissue cells, for repair of damage, or both. All these cells need a good supply of oils to build their cell walls, and the body keeps them handy. Every lymph gland in the body (such as the glands that get enlarged in your neck when you have a throat infection, precisely because they are the local headquarters for the immune system) carries a pad of fat around it—food for when it needs to produce white cells in a hurry. And the intestines, which are always "a busy immunological organ," carry an adjacent fat store in the omentum. The more inflammation in the gut, the bigger the belly. Food intolerances, of course, can be a major cause of gut inflammation; that's why so many people with intolerances can't lose weight on slimming diets, but really do when they identify and cut out their "bad" foods.

Polyunsaturated fats have a lower melting point, so they stay liquid (that is, they don't freeze) down to a lower temperature. That's why cold-water fish are so rich in polyunsaturates, and why an analysis of the lipid composition of the tissues of reindeer, which spend a lot of time standing in snow, showed that they have an increasing level of polyunsaturates as you go down the leg toward the hoof—so, the nearer the ground, the more resistant to freezing are the cells. Cell walls need to stay semi-liquid in order to move and to do all the things they do, and they need the polyunsaturates to keep them like that.

But if they are too liquid, they will lose their structure and fall apart. It's a tight balance that has to be maintained, and cholesterol and saturated fats are the molecules that provide the structure and solidity. Despite all you hear, it's actually having a *lower* cholesterol level that is linked to more illness and death, including heart disease, cancer, mental illness, and infections.[35]

Take a look at the composition of a normal cell wall:

- Polyunsaturated fats, 33 percent

- Saturated fats, 32 percent

- Cholesterol, 32 percent

If the structures that actually define life are composed of one third each of polyunsaturated oil, saturated oil, and cholesterol, how can any of them be bad for you? We need them all. A low-fat or low-cholesterol diet deprives you of them, and a junk food diet replaces them with unnecessary, undesirable things like trans-fats.

THE PROBLEM WITH TRANS-FATS

There is one real villain in all this: trans-fats. These are produced when unsaturated fats are hydrogenated (hydrogen atoms are artificially added). When you read on a label that a product contains "partially hydrogenated vegetable oil," it means that the unsaturated fats have been converted to trans-fats. The purpose of doing this is that it makes fats more solid at room temperature and less prone to going rancid, so they don't need refrigeration and have a longer shelf life. One of their biggest uses is in shortening, the oil used in much baking, which gives crispness and crumble to cookies and the like. Some shortenings, made from soy oil or rapeseed oil, contain 40–50 percent trans-fats. The irony is that the more polyunsaturates in the oil to begin with, the more trans-fats in the finished product.

The problem with trans-fats is that we don't have the enzymes to deal with them, so they hang around in the body much longer, clogging up our cell walls, our metabolism, and, it seems, our arteries. Ordinary fats are burned for energy, but we just can't break down and burn trans-fats. The risk of heart disease doubles with just a 2 percent increase in the trans-fats component of diet,[36] which is a far bigger effect than with any other lipid.

The evidence is mounting that trans-fats increase your risk of the following:

- Obesity and Diabetes—Both trans-fats or overall increased fat intake in general contribute to obesity and diabetes.

- Infertility—A 2 percent increase in trans-fats intake increased the risk of infertility by a staggering 73 percent in one study.[37]

- Cardiovascular Heart Disease—A thorough review in the *New England Journal of Medicine* concluded that "trans-fats appear to increase the risk of CHD more than any other macronutrient, conferring a substantially increased risk at low levels of consumption (1 to 3 percent of total energy intake)."[38]

- Cancer—Studies have shown a connection between trans-fat intake and breast[39] and prostate[40] cancers.

- Alzheimer's Disease—While trans-fats are by no means the only factor in Alzheimer's, they are an important one.[41]

Although there is a little trans-fat in dairy products, it doesn't seem to cause any problems, because its composition is not exactly the same as the "synthetic" trans-fats, so our bodies can use it. Most of it is in the form of conjugated linoleic acid (CLA). Although this is a trans-fat in a way, it's a form that our bodies can use and it appears to be beneficial, reducing the risk of obesity, diabetes, heart disease, and cancer.[42] Or at least some of it does; there are two major forms of CLA: one occurs naturally in beef and dairy products and is linked to all these benefits, while the other has been linked to some detrimental effects. Right now, I wouldn't advise taking CLA supplements. I would recommend eating its natural sources: the meat of ruminant animals (beef, lamb, venison), dairy products, and eggs. The meat has more CLA if it is reared naturally and free range, because then the animal is grass-fed rather than eating prepared feedstuffs.

Omega-3 versus Omega-6

There are two types of essential (which means you have to get them from food) polyunsaturated fats, omega-6 and omega-3. Omega-3s are found in fish oil; omega-6s come mainly from plants (vegetables, beans, nuts). There has been a lot of research on the health benefits of omega-3s, with many papers suggesting that eating more may reduce your risk of cancer, heart disease, and immune disorders, and improve brain function. But other studies have found no such benefit, and the reason is plain—you need both of them for normal healthy function. Just as cutting right down on your overall fat intake can be a bad thing, so can cutting down your omega-6s in favor of omega-3s.

There is one circumstance in which a high omega-3 intake, including supplements, can show a rapid dramatic benefit—in children with attention deficit/hyperactivity disorder (ADHD), autism, and other problems of neurodevelopment. Sometimes, but not always, putting a kid with these kinds of problems on omega-3 supplements enables them to leap forward in just a month or so. The reason, probably, is that the longer-chain omega-3s, especially docosahexaenoic acid (DHA), are important building blocks of nerve cells, so you need enough of them to build all the nerve cells that the growing brain needs. And if they are not needed, taking a supplement for up to three months certainly won't do any harm, so it's worth a try. There are studies that suggest the same pattern of response in adult depression.[43]

A number of scientific studies have looked at the anti-inflammatory effect of omega-3s, which is undeniably real. They damp down inflammation, which is why they can have an effect in heart disease and autoimmune diseases such as rheumatoid arthritis. However, too much omega-3s for too long can make you run short of omega-6s. These are generally described as being "pro-inflammatory," which is broadly true and which is generally considered to be a bad thing—but it's not that simple. Your body activates inflammation to produce an immune response or for repair of tissue damage, which is what the fat stores are needed for. No fats means no inflammation, no immune response, no healing.

The omega-6s are the important ones for inflammation, especially one called arachidonic acid. It's this molecule more than any other which is converted by the body into the short-term messenger molecules called prostaglandins. There are lots of these messengers (hormones, of a sort) and they can have different effects: some cause bronchoconstriction (tightening of the tubes of the lung), others cause bronchodilatation (loosening). They are all made from omega-6s, although arachidonic acid is the main one.

All allergy involves inflammation, and you want to regulate that inflammation but not switch it off, which would block the healing.

NSAIDS AND INFLAMMATION

The conversion of fatty acids, particularly arachidonic acid, into prostaglandins is done by an enzyme called cyclo-oxygenase (COX), and it is this enzyme that is blocked by aspirin and all the other NSAIDs (nonsteroidal, anti-inflammatory drugs) used as painkillers and inflammation suppressors. All of them can have the adverse effect of making stomach ulcers worse, and they can even cause bleeding from the ulcer and perforation of the bowel. Why? Because they block the healing effects of arachidonic acid and the omega-6s.

That was why the COX-2 inhibitors were introduced: remember Vioxx and Celebrex? Two of the best-selling drugs of the last decade, they turned out to have serious cardiovascular side effects, which outweighed their reduced (but not abolished) rate of gut side effects. When Vioxx was pulled from the market, it was estimated to have caused up to 55,000 deaths in the U.S.[44] Some scientists talked about "silent inflammation" occurring when the normal pathways are blocked by NSAIDs. Hiding the symptoms without treating the causes can be a *very* bad idea.

Dose

Donald Rudin, author of *Omega-3 Oils: A Practical Guide,* was a Harvard professor, a physician, and a mathematician. He was one of the first to experiment with a high omega-3 intake (from flax oil), and he found that it could improve the symptoms of eczema, psoriasis, many bowel disorders, and a list of other inflammatory problems. But the benefit only lasted for around three months, after which the symptoms returned. If his patients then stopped taking the flax oil, they got better again. Months later, the symptoms usually returned, so he restarted them on the flax oil diet and they improved again, for a while.

There's only one reasonable explanation for this two-way response—you need a balance. Too much or too little of either omega-3s or omega-6s is bad, while the right ratio of the two is good. So what is the right combination? It's tricky to answer that, but not impossible. Various studies have suggested the following ratios of omega-6 to omega-3 dietary intake for specific diseases[45]:

- Asthma, 5:1

- Cardiovascular disease, 4:1

- Cancers, 2.5:1

- Rheumatoid arthritis, 2:1 to 3:1

A "typical" American diet is said to have a 10:1 ratio, although some have calculated it as high as 30:1. Obviously, that deprives you of omega-3s (as well as giving you lots of trans-fats). But a high intake of omega-3s (taking lots of fish oil for a long time, for instance) can block your omega-6s. In fact, it seems that a too-high intake of either oil can suppress the metabolism of them both.

So, different diseases respond to different ratios, but is there a middle way that works for them all? The solution was worked out by a team of scientists in Israel and America, and it's not based on what ratio is best for any disease but on the best ratio for absorbing both kinds of oil. It's simple: consume them in the ratio of 4:1 omega-6 to omega-3.[46] This ratio, both in food and in supplements, will give you the best absorption of both types, the best metabolism of them into their destination molecules, and the best clinical effects on brain function, cardiovascular health, and immune function.

An anti-allergy diet can help you get the correct ratio of omega-3s and omega-6s to regulate inflammation. The diet, in fact, is the same one as we should eat for all sorts of health reasons: regular fish, but not too much; regular meat, dairy products, and eggs, but not too much; and *lots* of vegetables (green leafy ones), grains, and nuts and seeds. The World Health Organization and many scientists used to recommend five portions of colored (green, red, yellow) vegetables and fruits daily; now they are mostly recommending 9–10 portions. While many people think that is because of the vitamins and cofactors in them, in fact the oils are just as important.

You could call this a semi-vegetarian diet. Vegetarians who also eat eggs and/or dairy products are unlikely to run into trouble; strict vegans are advised to take a supplement derived from plant sources. If you have an allergy, or indeed any health problem that involves inflammation, take a 4:1 supplement in addition to the diet, at least until your health improves.

Guidelines

- For prevention, eat lots of green and other colored vegetables, fruits, nuts and seeds; some oily fish for the omega-3s; and some meat, eggs, and dairy products for the omega-6s.

- Stay away from processed foods that may contain trans-fats.

- For treating a health problem, also take a supplement: oils with an omega-6 to omega-3 ratio of around 4:1.

MAGNESIUM

While there's not a lot of scientific evidence that magnesium helps allergies in general, there *is* good evidence that injected magnesium is as useful as bronchodilating drugs at helping acute asthma,[47] and one paper showed that it helps nearly 50 percent of patients with chemical sensitivities.[48] However, magnesium is central to many processes in the body, and most of us are deficient in it, so there are good reasons to expect it to work for allergies. My personal clinical experience is that it does help.

The two minerals calcium and magnesium operate rather like the accelerator and the brakes in our cells. Calcium makes cells do what they do—muscles contract, blood vessels constrict, nerves discharge. Magnesium makes cells return to the "resting state." An excess of calcium has the same effect as a lack of magnesium— giving cells a hair trigger. This imbalance is central to over-reactivity of cells, which can lead to symptoms such as anxiety, jumpiness, muscle cramps, muscle twitching and tics, raised blood pressure, irregular heartbeat, angina, asthma, headaches, insomnia, ADHD, and seizures.

Magnesium can help all of these symptoms and has been doing so for decades. It is the key ingredient in Epsom salts; if you've ever sat in an Epsom salt bath to relax and ease tired muscles, you were taking a dose of magnesium (absorbed through the skin). When absorbed, it relaxes the blood vessels and the muscles and so allows the toxic metabolites, such as lactic acid, to flow away in the blood (lactic acid is what gives you the pain, or burn, in muscles when you overwork them). Muscle over-reactivity, or just plain overactivity, produces exhaustion. When your muscle cells are on a hair trigger, they do several times more work, contracting and relaxing rapidly, than a smoothly functioning muscle. So they burn up more energy, and overactivity leads to muscle fatigue. This is one reason why magnesium deficiency leads to fatigue.

Magnesium is also important for the energy supply inside cells.

Energy is produced by the mitochondria, the microscopic "batteries" in cells, in the form of a molecule called ATP (adenosine triphosphate). Each ATP molecule is delivered with an atom of magnesium; if you don't have enough magnesium, your mitochondria can't deliver enough energy to the cell. Now, it would be too simplistic to suggest that this *only* leads to the symptom of fatigue, or lack of energy. For example, in the brain there are cells that stimulate and cells that regulate or sedate. If the latter are the ones affected by lack of energy, you don't get fatigue but rather overactivity, and potentially all the symptoms listed above. But lack of energy supply certainly does lead to fatigue; a 2009 study on chronic fatigue patients showed that almost every one of them had a problem with mitochondrial energy supply.[49]

Studies show that if you have a classical, histamine-based allergy, and you're also deficient in magnesium, you will react more severely to exposure to an allergen.[50] In other words, magnesium appears to counteract histamine, the main initiator in allergies. If you're short of magnesium, there are several reasons why your allergy symptoms may be worse. In inhalant allergies, the reaction in the lungs will be worse: magnesium protects against asthma according to one large survey,[51] and intravenous magnesium is as good as salbutamol at turning asthma off.[52]

Magnesium is helpful for a long list of other disorders and diseases, including fatigue, anxiety and panic attacks (it calms down the hair trigger), muscle cramps and spasms (it relaxes the muscles), headaches and migraines (it relaxes the blood vessels), heart disease (relieves angina, reduces the damage from heart attack, and lowers blood pressure), circulation problems, and gynecological problems (PMS, menstrual cramps, and preeclampsia). I could add constipation as well, because surgeons often give a megadose of magnesium to clear out the gut before an operation (a "bowel prep"). It's designed to be far more than the body can absorb, so it stays in the bowel, attracts water to itself and gives you watery bowel motions. If you take too much magnesium yourself, it can do the same.

Dose

For an adult, the amount of magnesium in your diet that is just enough to keep your blood and tissue levels normal is usually around 300–600 mg per day. The amount that is more than your body can absorb, so it will give you loose bowels, is probably 800–1,200 mg. So, if you double your magnesium intake suddenly, you could jump straight from too little to too much without ever passing through the good zone. A day or two of loose bowels won't do you any harm, though, as long as you recognize it for what it is and act accordingly. This only applies to what you take by mouth, of course. For other routes of intake, you need a doctor in the loop to make sure that you don't take the wrong amount. We use magnesium by intravenous or intramuscular injection and by inhalation from a nebulizer.

A magnesium bath is another good option, and lots of people find this helpful. On their own, magnesium baths won't correct your deficiency, but alongside oral supplements they are a useful addition. Take a big handful of Epsom salts, which you can buy at the pharmacy, and stir it into a reasonably hot bath, full enough to cover you up to the neck. Spend at least 15 minutes in the bath. Repeat two or three times per week. If you have a chemical sensitivity, avoid proprietary Epsom salts brands with added scents or other ingredients; you can safely use generic Epsom salts without additives.

Guidelines

- Most of us need magnesium, so it's worth a try.

- Use baths as well as oral supplementation to boost your levels.

- You don't have to take it more than once a day, but it usually works better that way.

- To take things further (to check your levels, to get injections, and to monitor the effect of treatment), you will need a doctor's assistance.

- Loose bowels means you've overdosed—reduce your intake level, don't stop it.

CHAPTER 7

EXERCISE AND LIFESTYLE CHANGES

EXERCISE

How much exercise do you get? Even if you've got a gym membership or a favorite sport, there's not many of us who get enough regular, steady exercise. According to researchers, 78 percent of Americans do not get an adequate amount of physical activity.[1] But regular exercise is what we were built for, except that we used to call it "work." The human body, with its long, strong legs and a broad back, was designed for walking and running, for carrying, for digging, and for working with tools. This is how humans lived up until recent history. World War Two changed everything, bringing in labor-saving devices, nuclear power, and many of the advances we take for granted now. Since then, our physical workload has diminished and we take in too many food calories as fuel for doing it. That's why we are all getting fatter.

But exercise isn't only good for losing weight or improving your body shape—it has a number of other benefits.

The Benefits of Exercise

- Exercise burns calories, but even if it doesn't have that effect for you, it can still reduce your risk of type 2 diabetes, which in turn helps everything work a little better, including your immune system.

- Exercise strengthens the heart, opens up the blood vessels and reduces high blood pressure, and helps your cardiovascular system stay fit as you get older.

- Exercise improves the blood flow and oxygen supply to your brain and helps to make new nerve cells, which improves learning, slows brain aging, and delays or prevents dementia.

- Exercise improves mood, lifts depression, and stimulates the release of endorphins, the natural "feel good" chemicals inside the brain that also help against addictions and have generally good effects on immunity and inflammation.

- Exercise counteracts chronic stress, lowering levels of the stress hormone cortisol. We all need cortisol for our immediate response to injuries, threats, and both physical and psychological stresses. But if chronic stress causes chronically raised cortisol levels, this can suppress the healing of injured tissues, block the brain's ability to learn, and impair the immune system's response.

- Exercise gives you what amounts to an abdominal massage via the diaphragm and the muscles of the abdomen and spine, stimulating the bowel and other abdominal organs, and encouraging healthy elimination of waste matter. Detoxification is something our bodies have to do every day—much more so now than 100 years ago due to all the artificial chemicals around us—and every bit helps.

- Exercise pushes more blood through the kidneys, helping elimination of waste by that route. At the same time, it increases sweating, which is also essential for detoxification.

- Exercise reduces chronic inflammation, which is an important part of allergies, as it is of heart disease, cancer, and practically everything that can go wrong with a human body.

- Finally, if you exercise outdoors, it exposes you to sunshine, which allows the body to manufacture vitamin D.

I haven't forgotten about allergies. While this list of the effects of exercise covers the whole body, *all* of them end up influencing the immune system for the better. Scientists now talk about psychoneuroimmunology—the idea that the brain, nerves, the glands, and digestion are all connected to the immune system; there is multi-way cross-talk between each of these organs and systems. The hip bone surely is connected to the thigh bone, and what goes on in one part of the body inevitably influences what happens in the rest of it. If you've ever had depression, you know what I'm talking about: it doesn't just make you feel sad or blue, rather it is a whole-body experience. Allergies, just like fatigue or constipation, are made better or worse by all the other things going on in the body and mind, and exercise is a fundamental because our bodies were made to be used.

How to Get Started Exercising

You can have too much of a good thing. You may have firsthand experience of falling ill through exhaustion, and there have been reports that marathon runners run an increased risk of infections because *too much* exercise can suppress the immune system. But common sense is a useful guide here, so let's draw up some guidelines.

Start small and build up—If you suddenly start pounding the pavement after a lifetime as a couch potato, then your joints would soon be screaming in painful protest; they're just not trained for that. In fact, your muscles, ligaments, lungs, and heart would all feel it, and the injuries could even stop you from exercising altogether, so you end up worse off. But you do need to push yourself a bit when exercising or you'll never progress. So start with what you know you can handle, and build on it by 10–25 percent every few days. If in doubt, get a fitness assessment at a gym.

All at once or little-and-often?—In between, actually. The evidence is complicated and not completely clear, but it suggests that you need at least 2–3 hours of exercise per week. And that less than 30 minutes at a stretch doesn't do as much good, at least for some purposes. So, at one extreme, running a marathon once a week won't do it (and may harm your joints and muscles), while at the other end, walking just 10 minutes to work in the morning and the same in the evening won't be enough to make a difference. Both of these types of exercise are fine as part of the mix (and a mix is good), but you do need to put aside some time for exercising several times a week.

Intense enough to get you sweating—There are so many arguments about the proper level of exercise intensity. If you ask at your gym, they may give you a formula based on your heart rate and your age. But if you don't want to be a gym bunny and just want to feel better and improve your allergies, then exercise enough to get a sweat going. This should be the right level to do you good. This was what was shown to work in the Nurses' Health Study to prevent diabetes.[2] And yes, *strenuous* gardening or *heavy* housework (not just a little light dusting) count as exercise.

SUNLIGHT

You can get a double benefit if your exercising is done in the open air, because you can also get some sunlight on your skin. We are constantly told that sunlight is dangerous, that it can give us skin cancer and wrinkles, and that we should avoid it. But in the last few years, more research is showing that sunlight is necessary for health and that it is good for us. Confused? You're entitled to be. Let's untie this knot and make some sense of it all.

The basic fact is that without sunlight there would be no life on Earth. Nutrition researcher and dentist Weston A. Price (1870–1948) once said, "The dinner we have eaten was a part of the sun but a few months ago." True, because sunlight provides the energy for photosynthesis in plants. Plants use this for their everyday energy supply and also to take the carbon from carbon dioxide to make all the molecules they need. Yes, that's "carbon capture," the natural kind. Photosynthesis worldwide traps about six times as much energy as the human race uses, in burning fossil fuels, in nuclear reactors, everything.

But it isn't only plants that have evolved to take advantage of sunlight—all animals, including humans, do so as well, and not just by eating the plants. The single biggest benefit we get from sunlight is vitamin D, which is made in the skin by an effect of ultraviolet (UV) light (the light that your sunscreen is designed to block). Except that with life and work moving increasingly indoors in recent times, and with scientists telling us to avoid the sun, most of us don't get nearly enough vitamin D. Even in sunny Australia, the result of their "Slip, Slap, Slop" sun protection campaign has been widespread vitamin D deficiency.

Even though there are some other factors that we know we get from sunlight, and no doubt others as well, vitamin D is probably the biggest wasted resource in public health. Because vitamin D doesn't only strengthen your bones and prevent osteoporosis, it also benefits you in a number of ways.

Dangers of Sun Exposure

Now, I'm not saying that sunlight doesn't contribute to skin cancer or to skin aging, but it is more complicated than that. Heavy lifetime exposure to sunlight does increase the risk of the most common cancers of skin, such as the little rodent ulcers and other forms that many people experience. These are the least dangerous forms of cancer that you can get, mainly because they are easy to spot early and to treat. You have at least a 95 percent chance of being alive five years after being diagnosed with one of these types of cancer.[3] The more dangerous form of skin cancer, melanoma, is often said also to be due to the sun, but if this is true, then it is a *sunburn* and not a suntan that's dangerous. A sunburn is a much bigger problem for people with a Celtic skin type (ginger hair, freckles, burn easily, and hardly tan).[4] Still, the five-year survival rate for melanoma overall is 91 percent.

As for skin aging, that's got as much to do with nutrition as

with sunlight, but it's also an issue mainly for the face. Getting
vitamin D and other benefits from sunlight depends on the skin
area exposed to the sun, and since the head is less than 10 percent
of skin surface area, you don't really need it. So protect it—wear
a hat, and if necessary, a good, more natural sunscreen. But get
your vitamin D by wearing short-sleeved shirts and shorts when
you can.

Skin Type and Sun Exposure

Some people aren't designed for the sun, specifically those with
ginger hair and freckles who never tan—they only go red and then
white again. This is known as type I skin, or Celtic skin, and it's
very different from the rest of us (see table "Skin Types and Sun
Sensitivity"). Scientists reckon this sort of skin evolved as mankind
moved into the frozen, or just thawed, far north of Europe, as a
way of catching as much of the scarce UV rays there as possible.
If that's your skin type, you have twice the risk of melanoma that
the rest of us have, and you should be very careful.

Apart from those with type I skin, everybody produces a pig-
ment called melanin in their skin in response to sunlight. Melanin
is what makes you tan. Those with type VI skin produce a lot more
melanin than those with type II, even when they don't get out in
the sun. People with type I skin produce a different kind of
melanin that doesn't show as a tan and doesn't protect from the
UV rays. The "exposure factor" means that a person with type VI
skin, for example, will need seven times as much sun to make them
burn as a type I person. So if a type I person is in Florida, where
the UV index can reach extremely high, they can probably only
handle 10 minutes in the sun before they start to burn, but a type
VI person can manage 70 minutes.

So getting enough sun to make vitamin D doesn't really apply
if you have type I skin. You should probably just take vitamin D
supplements instead (see Chapter 6). As for the rest of us, the sun
is there for a reason. Make the most of it, but be sensible—tan,

SKIN TYPES AND SUN SENSITIVITY				
SKIN TYPE	ETHNIC GROUP	APPEARANCE	SENSITIVITY TO SUN	EXPOSURE FACTOR
I	Celtic	White skin, freckles, blue eyes, red or blond hair	Burn very easily; do not tan	1
II	Nordic	Pale skin, freckles, blue or hazel eyes, red or blond hair	Burn easily; tan slowly and slightly	1.5
III	Most "white" people	Fair skin, blond or brunette	Brown moderately; tan slowly and moderately	2
IV	Mediterranean, Chinese/Japanese, Amerindian	Olive or light brown skin, dark hair, dark eyes	Burn slightly; tan easily	2.5
V	Arab, Malaysian, Mexican, Indian	Brown skin, hair and eyes brown or black	Burn rarely; tan well and deeply	3.5
VI	Black, Aborigine, Melanesian	Skin brown to black, hair and eyes black	Never burn; remain dark-skinned	7

Source: Weller, R., J. Hunter, J. Savin, et al. *Clinical Dermatology,* 4th ed. Malden, MA: Blackwell, 2008.

don't burn. And if you can't get out in the sun, you should take a vitamin D supplement too.

Guidelines

Little and often—Sunning so much that you burn gives you no advantage and carries risks. Getting enough sun to just start to tan is enough for the vitamin D effect. And you need this regularly throughout the year, not just a once-a-year blitz.

Know your skin type and act on it—If your skin is type I, be very careful. Any other skin type, figure out how much sun is safe for you and never exceed that on any one day.

Enjoy—The sun is a natural gift and is meant to be a pleasure, so make the most of it. Regard it with respect but not fear.

CHAPTER 8

DESENSITIZATION AND OTHER OPTIONS

What can you do if none of the previously discussed options work? While it's my experience with several thousand patients that these natural solutions work, there's always one person for whom nothing seems to work. Let it not be you, but if it is, here are some other options.

DESENSITIZATION

A vaccination is a small dose of something (an infection such as tetanus or meningitis) designed to make your immune system respond to it in future—to *sensitize* you. Desensitization involves a small dose of something (an allergen such as pollen or milk, for example) designed to stop your immune system from responding—to *desensitize* you. Whether these small doses have a sensitizing or desensitizing effect, or none, depends on the dose, what other chemicals and molecules are in the shot, and the route of administration.

A good example of the route of administration is what I said previously in the book about babies developing anaphylaxis to peanuts when they had never eaten it but had touched it. Touching it first meant they developed this violent allergic reaction; if they had eaten it first, they would almost certainly have tolerated it fine, as most people do. This shows how simply changing the point of contact with something can have a powerful effect.

Making that work for good rather than bad is what both vaccination and desensitization are trying to do.

The baby who is first exposed to peanut on the skin, before they ever eat it, and reacts to it also illustrates that a lot of immunity goes on in the skin, and that tiny doses can have very large effects. Several researchers have noted that as you dilute an allergen more and more, its effect on the body's response changes with each step. For instance, take pure milk and dilute 1 part of it with 4 parts of pure water and you have a 1-in-5 solution. Take 1 part of that and dilute it the same way and it's now a 1-in-25 solution. Repeat four more times, and you will have, lined up in a row, solutions of 1 in 125, 1 in 625, 1 in 3,125, and 1 in 15,625. That's called serial dilution.

Now, take a drop of each of these in order, and put it under your tongue. If you don't have a problem with milk, nothing will happen, but if you're allergic to milk, each dose should have a different effect. Pure milk would probably make you feel quite bad, but as you try progressively higher dilutions (smaller doses) that will change, until you reach a dose that switches off your symptoms. That is known as the neutralizing dose, and the whole process of using this to control your symptoms is known as neutralization therapy.

If you keep doing serial dilution, and testing the resulting doses on your allergy, it seems that a couple or so doses after the first neutralizing dose the effect reverses. So it makes the symptoms worse, then reverses again and makes them better, and continues doing that as long as you keep diluting. If you keep doing it long enough—about forty times for the 1-in-5 doses—you will pass Avogadro's number, which is the point beyond which there should not be a single molecule left of the original solution. Then you're in the realm of homeopathy; remarkably, researchers have reported that the same thing keeps on happening.

The point about other molecules in the shot or in the drops under the tongue is also important. Vaccinations use what are called adjuvants, molecules in the mix that are intended to irritate, or activate, the immune system so that it will react, preferably to the virus or other infecting agent in the vaccine. Using other molecules, ones that occur naturally in the body, can help to persuade the immune system to accept (tolerate) allergens. That is the basis of another method of desensitization known as enzyme-potentiated desensitization (EPD). Let's look at these treatment methods.

Conventional Hyposensitization

Years ago, when I was a family doctor, I used to give patients this treatment, and then it was banned in the United Kingdom because of some deaths associated with it. The practice continued in the U.S., and has made a limited come-back in the U.K. in the last few years, though only in hospitals where all the gear is available to deal with an emergency. It is best described as "incremental" desensitization: you start at a low injected dose, and every week for around ten weeks you get a slightly bigger dose, in the hope that the immune system will be persuaded to accept or tolerate it. It certainly works sometimes, but in my opinion the rates are poor and it's not worth the risk and effort. Naturally, you will find doctors who disagree strongly with that view.

Neutralization

This technique was developed first in the 1950s by Dr. Carleton Lee, and then refined by Dr. Joseph Miller in Alabama, and described in print by him in 1972.[1] It starts with testing to find the "end-point" or neutralizing dose for each allergen. This can be done either by very small injections into the skin or with drops under the tongue. It takes time to test each food or other allergen one by one, usually between 20 and 60 minutes, so only a few can be tested in one session before both patient and tester have had enough. Once the end-points have been determined, a treatment is mixed up for you to use when needed, either by injection or under the tongue. This may need to be done anywhere between twice a week and several times a day. Sometimes the fact of treating the allergy seems to make the end-points shift and you have to go back for retesting.

There have been several studies that have claimed to show that neutralization doesn't work,[2] but each of them has had problems with its method. There are some small studies showing it is effective.[3] I studied it and took the course back in the 1980s, and I can say from experience that it often does work. I don't use it now, not because of any lack of efficacy, but because for a doctor it requires holding stock of every allergen you may need, and I wasn't doing enough treatments for that to be financially viable. It's certainly safe; I am aware of no serious adverse reactions either in published studies or experienced by colleagues. Minor reactions during testing are common, though.

My take on neutralization, and there are doctors who will disagree, is that:

- It is fast-acting, so you don't need to plan way ahead.

- But it's also short-acting, so you have to keep doing it.

- It is great for occasional use (say to something which you normally avoid but can't always), but used constantly, day in and day out, it tends to lose effectiveness.

- It is good for single allergies, or for just a few, but gets complicated and potentially expensive for lots of allergies.

- It is probably the most effective single treatment for symptoms of chemical sensitivity.

- However, it just doesn't work for some people, maybe one in twenty.

- It is definitely safe.

Enzyme-Potentiated Desensitization

EPD was developed by Dr. Len McEwen at St. Mary's Hospital in London, following a chance finding in the early 1960s that the naturally occurring enzyme beta-glucuronidase given before an exposure reduced the allergic symptoms. Dr. McEwen has spent the last forty years refining and improving the method, and it's still improving. I've been using it for twenty-five years.

The way it works is that all the allergens are mixed together in one vial, and the enzymes are in another vial; the two are mixed together immediately before giving it. We used to give it onto the skin, under a plastic cup, but now it's done by a very small injection (literally two or three drops) into the top layer of skin (intradermally). The doses of the allergens and enzymes have been carefully calculated and don't change. The enzymes are there to potentiate, or increase, the desensitizing effect. Injections are generally around one every three months, but that typically increases later to four, six, or even twelve months or more.

EPD doesn't need any testing for dose levels, but it certainly helps to know what the patient is allergic to, at least approximately, for two reasons. Firstly, because there are about five different mixes of allergens, and we need to decide which one is right for you. Secondly, because it's a very small dose, maybe a few thousand molecules of wheat or dairy; if you had some the day before the injection, there will be millions of molecules of it still in your system, which will swamp the tiny dose in the injection and prevent it from working. So you need to avoid eating your allergens around the time of the shot.

There have been nine controlled trials of EPD that have shown it to be effective,[4] and one that didn't.[5] Guess which study got all the publicity. That's a pretty good score in favor of it. I usually tell patients that it is successful in at least 80 percent of cases in general, although individual results may vary. It's only done in a clinical setting, where we have all the necessary treatments should something go wrong. There have never been any deaths linked to EPD, and I have never heard of a severe reaction. In twenty-five years, I have only once gotten to the stage of drawing up an epinephrine shot in case I needed it in a hurry; I did not use it.

There were once about 200 doctors in the United States and Canada using EPD, until the U.S. Food and Drug Administration stepped in and closed it down. To keep it alive in the U.S., the former head of the American EPD Society got together with a compounding pharmacy and produced low-dose allergotherapy. It is similar to EPD and has about the same success rate.

EPD, in summary, is characterized by the following:

- It is slow-acting, so you do need to plan well ahead (for summer rhinitis, for instance, you need to start treatment three months in advance).

- It is cumulative and long-lasting, so you may be able to stop treatment after several years. Also, you need to be prepared to commit to at least two years of treatment at the start.

- It's best for multiple allergies, especially to a combination of foods/inhalants/chemicals.

- It is also good for preventing bad reactions to insect bites and for yeast allergies and reactions to other organisms.

- Most people need to follow a strict diet around the time of treatments, and they often take certain medications (such as antifungal drugs) and/or supplements to improve the success rate.

OTHER COMPLEMENTARY METHODS

Leaving aside allergy testing methods such as applied kinesiology, there are two other treatment methods to consider.

Homeopathic Desensitization

Most homeopathic remedies are intended to address the person's constitution, to treat the deep causes of disease within them. Whether constitutional homeopathy works is a big subject—I've seen it work and I've seen it fail. Homeopathic desensitization is frowned on by some homeopaths because it uses dilutions of the food or other allergen, not a constitutional remedy. It, too, does work sometimes; since it is cheap and relatively harmless, if you want to try it I say go ahead. You should be able to figure out whether it is any use in a matter of weeks at most, and if not you can then turn to another option, such as desensitization.

NAET

Nambudripad's Allergy Elimination Technique (NAET) was developed by a chiropractor, Devi Nambudripad, who personally had experienced numerous food intolerances. She found that using treatments such as acupressure *when in contact with an allergen* could block that allergy. Does it work? I'm aware of no formal study, but there are certainly many people who say it has helped them. Is it safe? I can't say for sure, but probably yes. Is it worth a try? Sure.

MEDICATIONS

I'm not sure that desensitization addresses the root cause of allergies. After all, the root cause may be in your genes, and we still can't do much about them. But taking medications for your allergies certainly won't do more than control the symptoms. That can be very useful, though, and I'm not saying you shouldn't do it; just be aware of the downside, which could include numerous and serious side effects. Vitamin C is still the most useful thing to quickly turn off most reactions, but there are two categories of drugs that can also help. The reason vitamin C is so helpful is that it is the body's natural defense against excess histamine.

Antihistamines

The earliest of antihistamines were, and still are, also useful as sedatives or tranquillizers. In other words, they can damp down both the immune system and the nervous system. In fact, the chemical group includes drugs like chlorpromazine (Thorazine, used to calm down psychotic patients), promethazine (used as a premed before surgery to stop you vomiting), and perphenazine (used for allergies). Since then, there have been several generations of new antihistamines, because they are useful and popular. Because they work both on the nervous system and on the rest of the body, they tend to make you sleepy (although the newer drugs are better in this regard). If you need to drive, this can be a serious downside; in other circumstances, it could be an up-side if the patient is not you but a whiney, unhappy child, for instance.

There's nothing to stop you from combining antihistamines with nutrients; in fact, this can be a useful approach. Just try the nutrients first, because I would sooner you took regular doses of nutrients and topped up when necessary with antihistamines than that you took the maximum dose of antihistamines plus the occasional supplement.

Steroids

Your body produces steroids (cortisol is the main one) to help deal with stress. Bear in mind that physical stresses can be much more important than psychological ones, although you won't be aware of them at the time. Pain, cold, heat, injury—they all cause the body to pump out cortisol. So does fear, anxiety, and worry; the problem is that these psychological stresses are liable to stick around and become chronic. We were designed to handle short-term physical threats, not the constant worry of negative equity or job loss.

Cortisol is designed to divert the body's energy where it is needed to deal with life's challenges, large and small (there's a little boost of cortisol to help you get up in the morning). That means diverting energy away from the immune system, which is why steroids are useful in allergies. One of the most popular for many years is a steroid called Kenalog, given as a single shot, before the pollen season starts, to control hay fever. The other major use has been steroid creams for eczema and other rashes.

The problem with steroids is that they work, but you have to keep on using them. Steroid creams will usually do a good job of controlling eczema, but once you stop the treatment the rash returns, so you go back on it and end up using it long-term. That's when the side effects begin. On the skin, the most obvious effect is steroid atrophy: the skin becomes smooth and featureless, with tiny blood vessels and bruising easily visible. This is very like premature aging of the skin and is usually not reversible. Just think what the effects of long-term use of steroid inhalers on the lung might be.

Steroids can save lives and that's a fact. My view is that they should be treated with the respect they deserve and kept for acute situations where they can really make a difference, not used every day for weeks on end. So if you do find yourself on long-term steroid treatment, keep trying to wean yourself off (under your doctor's supervision); the nutrients described in this book can help. And the same thing I said about antihistamines is true here: it's much better to take regular nutrients plus a steroid when really needed than the other way around.

CONCLUSION

We are in an epidemic of allergies—nobody would deny this. The reasons are many, but much of the evidence points to increasing levels of pollution and to sedentary lifestyles as major factors. There is a lot you can do to help yourself in those areas. But the single biggest reason that so many of us are getting to be allergic is diet and nutrition, for several reasons and in several ways.

Our diets have too many calories, and most of those calories are in the form of carbohydrates—sugar, white flour, and so on. There are also too many bad fats, the hydrogenated and trans-fats that are created in factories, not grown on farms. Both carbohydrates and trans-fats are known to interfere with our immune systems, to weaken our resistance to infections and at the same time make us more prone to allergies. Our diets are also short on many of the ingredients that are essential for life, the vitamins, minerals, and oils essential for a smoothly functioning immune system (not to mention a smoothly functioning brain, heart, and so on). Factory farming and food processing have taken so much of the goodness out of our food, but you really have to laugh at the absurdity of humanity putting itself on a low-fat diet. Every cell in your body has a wall of fats and oils around it—without oils, there would be no life on the planet. Deprive your body of them and it can't make new cells and thus can't repair itself. You will also deprive yourself of the fat-soluble vitamins, most importantly vitamin D, which we should be getting from sunlight, but mostly don't.

If you've got an allergy, what can you do to help yourself? Pharmaceutical drugs are helpful sometimes, but generally they only reduce the symptoms, and only if you keep taking them, for which there is often a price to pay in side effects. However, some allergies are life-threatening, and then the medications may be unavoidable and life-saving. If the symptom is that serious, then you have no choice but to stop it, by whatever means possible. Please don't imagine that I would ever ask you to refuse vital medication. But both in the potentially dangerous allergies and in the less dangerous ones, which can still make life truly miserable, there are *always* things you can do to help yourself.

The first step is knowledge: figure out what you are reacting to, and understand where it is coming from. Use this knowledge to avoid the allergen and cut it out of your diet or your environment as best you can. Then clean up your diet, your environment, and your lifestyle. Cut out the chemicals and the junk food; eat well and sensibly—and locally, if you can, for the sake of the planet. Plus, get out there and exercise.

But all of that is prevention. The one thing you can do that can both prevent *and* treat allergies is nutrition. You may well need to do this both through your diet and with supplements. The most important ones—the big four—are vitamin C, vitamin D, magnesium, and essential fatty acids. Once you understand something of how these work, and how to use them, then you can really help yourself.

I hope that by using the methods outlined in this book in your own life, you will find relief from your allergies.

RESOURCES

These days information isn't really information unless it is on the Internet. Patients often ask or tell their doctors about the results of their own Internet research. Medical journals get quite stuffy about this, saying that most of the information on the web is of poor quality and biased by commercial interests. They have a point, of course—if a website is trying to sell you something, they are unlikely to push, and may even suppress, negative information about it. After all, pharmaceutical companies have been caught repeatedly doing just that. In providing these links, I have therefore avoided commercial interests with two notable exceptions, both fully justifiable I believe.

Do your own research by all means, provided that you have a skeptical attitude and you are careful to recognize and acknowledge when you are out of your depth and need an expert to help you out. Then you should go find it under "Physicians" below.

ALLERGIES, GENERAL

Allergy UK
www.allergyuk.org
I don't know of a U.S.-based resource that I trust as much as Allergy UK, whose website has large amounts of information on allergies, treatments, and products (but U.K.-biased, of course).

Avon Study
www.bristol.ac.uk/alspac/

The Avon Longitudinal Study of Parents and Children (also known as Children of the '90s) has taught us some important insights about how and why allergies develop. The website summarizes findings for the nonmedical person.

ANAPHYLAXIS

Food Allergy and Anaphylaxis Alliance
www.foodallergyalliance.org

This group works to "unite organizations working in food allergy and anaphylaxis in order to exchange information, form partnerships, and advance key issues of importance to those with food allergy and anaphylaxis." In other words, it is the one-stop shop for information and support from organizations around the world.

Epipen
www.epipen.com

The Epipen Auto-Injector is the essential life-saving self-treatment for people with life-threatening allergies. It is only available by prescription; your doctor will know all about it.

AUTISM

Autism Research Institute
www.autism.com

The Autism Research Institute was founded in 1967. From then to the present day, it has been the most trustworthy source of information on what autism is really about.

CHEMICAL SENSITIVITIES

There are so many websites dealing with multiple chemical sensitivities (MCS) that it is difficult to know which to recommend. A lot of them are either commercially sponsored or are one-man bands, although neither automatically makes them unreliable. It is my personal opinion that these two are the best I know of:

Chemical Injury Information Network
www.ciin.org

Allergy UK's Chemical Sensitivity pages
www.allergyuk.org/art_mcs.aspx

National Center for Healthy Housing
www.nchh.org
The National Center for Healthy Housing campaigns, researches, and provides information and resources about a range of risks that can come from indoor factors in homes, including toxic mold, chemical pollutants, pests, and the pesticide treatments used for them.

FOOD

Slow Food

The Slow Food movement is a worldwide network that "links the pleasure of food with a commitment to community and the environment." They run campaigns in schools and colleges to educate about traditional, local, and sustainable foods.

Slow Food International
www.slowfood.com

Slow Food USA
www.slowfoodusa.org

Organic Center

www.organic-center.org

The Organic Center produces research, reports, guides, blogs, and links on the benefits of organic farming and food, how to go organic, and how to avoid pesticides in food.

MINERAL WATER

Mineral Waters of the World

www.mineralwaters.org

This extraordinary website lists, tastes, and provides sourcing information for over 3,000 mineral waters worldwide. They don't make unsound claims—for example, this is what they say about tap water: "Depending on where you live, the tap water may be drinkable, in some instances it is in fact very good. At many places, tap water has a composition similar to a still mineral water. . . . On the other hand, there are many countries where tap water is inherently unsafe to drink."

NUTRITIONAL THERAPY

Orthomolecular Medicine News Service

www.orthomolecular.org

The Orthomolecular Medicine News Service is run by Dr. Andrew Saul, who is the series editor for Basic Health's Vitamin Cure books, which includes this book. The OMNS works to "counter the pharmaceutically biased factoids and vitamin misinformation that the media so often accept uncritically" with readable, plain-speaking news releases that are sometimes funny too. (But I'm biased—I'm on the editorial board.)

Linus Pauling Institute

www.lpi.oregonstate.edu

The Linus Pauling Institute at Oregon State University runs a Micronutrient Information Center with lots of information on most vitamins, minerals, and other nutrients.

Vitamin D

GrassrootsHealth

www.grassrootshealth.net

The D*Action campaign at GrassrootsHealth provides news and information on vitamin D, plus a low-cost testing service as part of its ongoing research project.

Vitamin C

Vitamin C Foundation

www.vitamincfoundation.org

The Vitamin C Foundation website publishes articles, a forum, links, etc., all about vitamin C therapy.

AscorbateWeb

www.seanet.com/~alexs/ascorbate/

AscorbateWeb is a remarkable compendium of scientific articles on vitamin C, from the 1930s to the new millennium.

Magnesium

Magnesium Website

www.mgwater.com

Paul Mason has a vested interest in that he produces a mineral water that is rich in magnesium, but he certainly doesn't run the Magnesium Website for profit—it is the best resource I know of for scientific information on the importance of magnesium.

PHYSICIANS

American Academy of Allergy, Asthma and Immunology
www.aaaai.org

The American Academy of Allergy, Asthma, and Immunology repre-
sents doctors in mainstream allergy practice. Members are well-versed
in treating straightforward allergies with shots and medications, but
the Academy is noncommittal about chemical sensitivities.

American Academy of Environmental Medicine
www.aaemonline.org

Members of the American Academy of Environmental Medicine are
experienced in and responsive to chemical problems and to approach-
es to allergy such as the nutritional ones in this book.

REFERENCES

Introduction

1. U.S. Centers for Disease Control and Prevention. *National Health Interview Survey.* Available online at: www.cdc.gov/nchs/nhis.

Chapter 1: What is an Allergy?

1. Gilliland, F.D., Y.-F. Li, H. Gong, et al. "Glutathione s-transferases M1 and P1 Prevent Aggravation of Allergic Responses by Secondhand Smoke." *Am J Resp Crit Care Med* 174:12 (December 2006): 1335–1341.

2. Egger, J., C.M. Carter, J. Wilson, et al. "Is Migraine Food Allergy? A Double-blind, Controlled Trial of Oligoantigenic Diet Treatment." *Lancet* 2 (1983): 865–869.

3. McKeown-Eyssen, G., C. Baines, D. Cole, et al. "Case-control Studies of Genotypes in Multiple Chemical Sensitivity: *CYP2D, NAT1, NAT2, PON1, PON2,* and *MTHFR.*" *Int J Epidemiol* 33 (2004): 1–8.

4. Farrow, A., H. Taylor, K. Northstone, et al.; ALSPAC Study Team. "Symptoms of Mothers and Infants Related to Total Volatile Organic Compounds in Household Products." *Arch Environ Health* 58:10 (2003): 633–641.

Chapter 2: Allergies That Kill

1. Sampson, H.A. "Food Anaphylaxis." *Brit Med Bull* 56:4 (2000): 925–935.

2. Lack, G., D. Fox, K. Northstone, J. Golding; Avon Longitudinal Study of Parents and Children Study Team. "Factors Associated with the Development of Peanut Allergy in Childhood." *N Engl J Med* 348:11 (March 2003): 977–985.

3. McEwen, L.M., and P. Constantinopolous. "The Use of a Dietary and Antibacterial Regime in the Management of Intrinsic Allergy." *Ann Allergy* 28 (1970): 256–266.

4. National Heart, Lung, and Blood Institute. National Asthma Education and Prevention Program. "Expert Panel Report 3: Guidelines for the Diagnosis and Management of Asthma." Bethesda, MD: National Institutes of Health, 2007. Available online at: www.nhlbi.nih.gov/guidelines/asthma/asthgdln.pdf.

5. Joneja, J.M.V. "Oral Allergy Syndrome, Cross-reacting Allergens and Co-occurring Allergies." *J Nutr Environ Med* 9 (1999): 289–303.

Chapter 3: Avoiding Inhalants

1. Lewis, S.A., J.M. Corden, G.E. Forster, et al. "Combined Effects of Aerobiological Pollutants, Chemical Pollutants and Meteorological Conditions on Asthma Admissions and A & E Attendances in Derbyshire UK, 1993–96." *Clin Exp Allergy* 30 (2000): 1724–1732.

2. Mudarri, D., and W.J. Fisk. "Public Health and Economic Impact of Dampness and Mold." *Indoor Air* 17:3 (June 2007): 226–235.

3. Lieberman, A. "Explosion of Mold Cases in Homes, Workplaces and Occupational Medicine Practices." Presented at the 21st Annual Symposium on Man and His Environment in Health and Disease, Dallas, Texas, June 19–22, 2003. Rea, W.J., N. Didriksen, T.R. Simon, et al. "Effects of Toxic Exposure to Molds and Mycotoxins in Building-related Illnesses." *Arch Environ Health* 58:7 (2003): 399–405.

4. Curtis, L., A. Lieberman, M. Stark, et al. "Adverse Health Effects of Indoor Molds." *J Nutr Environ Med* 14:3 (2004): 261–274.

5. Sprott, T.J. "Cot Death-Cause and Prevention." *J Nutr Environ Med* 14:3 (2004): 221–235.

Chapter 4: Avoiding Foods and Chemicals

1. Pollan, M. *In Defense of Food.* New York: Penguin, 2008.

Chapter 5: Genes, Pollution, and Diet

1. Autism Research Institute (ARI). "Survey on Parent Ratings of Behavioural Effects of Biomedical Interventions." ARI Publication 34, 2008. Available online at: www.autism.com/treatable/form34qr.htm.

2. Gilliland, F.D., Y.-F. Li, H. Gong, D. Diaz-Sanchez. "Glutathione S-Transferases M1 and P1 Prevent Aggravation of Allergic Responses by Secondhand Smoke." *Am J Resp Crit Care Med* 174:12 (December 2006): 1335–1341.

3. Brasch-Andersen, C., L. Christiansen, Q. Tan, et al. "Possible Gene Dosage Effect of Glutathione-S-transferases on Atopic Asthma: Using Real-time PCR for Quantification of GSTM1 and GSTT1 Gene Copy Numbers." *Hum Mutat* 24:3 (September 2004): 208–214.

4. McKeown-Eyssen, G., C. Baines, D.E.C. Cole, et al. "Case-control Study of Geno-types in Multiple Chemical Sensitivity: CYP2D6, NAT1, PON1, PON2, and NTHFR." *Int J Epidemiol* 33:5 (2004): 1–8.

5. Schnakenberg, E., K.R. Fabig, M. Stanulla, et al. "A Cross-sectional Study of Self-reported Chemical-related Sensitivity is Associated with Gene Variants of Drug Metabolizing Enzymes." *Environ Health* 6 (February 2007): 6.

6. Mineralwaters.org. "Mineral Waters of the World." Available online at: www.mineral-waters.org.

7. Stapleton, H.M., S.M. Kelly, J.G. Allen, et al. "Measurement of Polybrominated Diphenyl Ethers on Hand Wipes: Estimating Exposure from Hand-to-Mouth Contact." *Environ Sci Technol* 42:9 (2008): 3329–3334

8. Holland, N., C. Furlong, M. Bastaki, et al. "Paraoxonase Polymorphisms, Haplotypes, and Enzyme Activity in Latino Mothers and Newborns." *Environ Health Perspect* 114:7 (2006): 985–991.

9. Rea, W. "Pesticides." *J Nutr Med* 6 (1996): 55–124.

10. Benbrook, C., X. Zhao, J. Yáñez, et al. "New Evidence Confirms the Nutritional Superiority of Plant-Based Organic Foods." The Organic Center, March 2008. Available online at: www.organic-center.org/reportfiles/5367_Nutrient_Content_SSR_FINAL_V2.pdf.

Chapter 6: Nutrition for Allergies

1. DiPasquale, D. "Magnesium Stearate: Terrible Toxin or Innocuous Additive?" *That's*

Fit. Available online at: www.thatsfit.ca/2009/04/29/magnesium-stearate-terrible-toxin-or-innocuous-additive/.

2. Pauling, L. "Ascorbic Acid and the Common Cold." *Am J Clin Nutr* 24:11 (1971): 1294–1299. Dahlberg, G., A. Engel, H. Rydin. "The Value of Ascorbic Acid as a Prophylactic Against Common Colds." *Acta Med Scand* (1944): 540–561. Dick, E.C., K.A. Mink, D. Olander, et al. "Amelioration of Rhinovirus Type 16 (RV16) Colds in Ascorbic Acid Supplemented Volunteers." 30th ICAC Proceedings, 1990. Anderson, T.W., G. Suranyi, G.H. Beaton. "The Effect on Winter Illness of Large Doses of Vitamin C." *Can Med Assoc J* 111 (1974): 31–36.

3. Pitt, H.A., and A.M. Costrini. "Vitamin C Prophylaxis in Marine Recruits." *JAMA* 241:9 (1979): 908–911. Gorton, H.C., and K. Jarvis. "The Effectiveness of Vitamin C in Preventing and Relieving the Symptoms of Virus-induced Respiratory Infections." *J Manipulat Physiol Ther* 8 (1999): 530–533. Magne, R.V. "Vitamin C in Treatment of Influenza." *El Dia Med* 35 (1963): 1714–1715.

4. Singh, P., et al. "Association Between Breast Cancer and Vitamin C, Vitamin E and Selenium Levels: Results of a Case-control Study in India." *Asian Pac J Cancer Prev* 6:2 (2005): 177–180. Yuan, J.M., et al. "Diet and Breast Cancer in Shanghai and Tianjin, China." *Br J Cancer* 71:6 (1995): 1353–1358. Enstrom, J.E., L.E. Kanim, M.A. Klein. "Vitamin C Intake and Mortality Among a Sample of the United States Population." *Epidemiology* 3:3 (May 1992): 194–202.

5. Cameron, E., and L. Pauling. "Supplemental Ascorbate in the Supportive Treatment of Cancer: Prolongation of Survival Times in Terminal Human Cancer." *Proc Natl Acad Sci U S A* 73:10 (1976): 3685–3689.

6. Hoffer, A. "Antioxidant Nutrients and Cancer." *J Orthomolecular Med* 15:4 (2000): 193–200.

7. Enstrom, J.E., L.E. Kanim, M.A. Klein. "Vitamin C Intake and Mortality Among a Sample of the United States Population." *Epidemiology* 3:3 (May 1992): 194–202.

8. Bucca, C., G. Rolla, et al. "Effect of Vitamin C on Histamine Bronchial Responsiveness of Patients with Allergic Rhinitis." *Ann Allergy* 65 (1990): 311–314. Hochwald, A. "Vitamin C in the Treatment of Croupous Pneumonia." *Deutsche Med Wochenschr* 63:5 (1937): 182–184.

9. Robin Harris, J. *Ascorbic Acid: Biochemistry and Biomedical Cell Biology.* New York: Plenum Press, 1996.

10. Holmes, Alexander, 1942.

11. Ruskin, 1947.

12. Hickey, S., H.J. Roberts, et al. "Pharmacokinetics of Oral Vitamin C." Publication pending.

13. Taylor, E.N., M.J. Stampfer, G.C. Curhan. "Dietary Factors and the Risk of Incident Kidney Stones in Men: New Insights after 14 Years of Follow-up." *J Am Soc Nephrol* 15:12 (2004): 3225–3232.

14. Linus Pauling Institute; Oregon State University. "Vitamin C." Available online at: lpi.oregonstate.edu/infocenter/vitamins/vitaminC/index.html.

15. "Effectiveness and Safety of Vitamin D in Relation to Bone Health." (Structured Abstract.) Rockville, MD: Agency for Healthcare Research and Quality, 2007. Available online at: www.ahrq.gov/clinic/tp/vitadtp.htm.

16. Turner, M.K., W.M. Hooten, J.E. Schmidt, et al. "Prevalence and Clinical Correlates of Vitamin D Inadequacy Among Patients with Chronic Pain." *Pain Med* 9:8 (November 2008): 979–984.

17. Garland, C.F., F.C. Garland, et al. "The Role of Vitamin D in Cancer Prevention." *Am J Public Health* 96 (2005): 252–261.

18. Aloia, J.F., and M. Li-Ng. "Epidemic Influenza and Vitamin D." *Epidemiol Infect* 135 (2007): 1095–1096.

19. Gloth 3rd, F.M., W. Alam, B. Hollis. "Vitamin D vs Broad-spectrum Phototherapy in the Treatment of Seasonal Affective Disorder." *J Nutr Health Aging* 3:1 (1999): 5–7.

20. Michos, E.D., and M.L. Melamed. "Vitamin D and Cardiovascular Disease Risk." *Curr Opin Clin Nutr Metab Care* 11:1 (January 2008): 7–12. Nemerovski, C.W., M.P. Dorsch, et al. "Vitamin D and Cardiovascular Disease." *Pharmacotherapy* 29:6 (June 2009): 691–708.

21. Pilz, S., H. Dobnig, et al. "Low Vitamin D Levels Predict Stroke in Patients Referred to Coronary Angiography." *Stroke* 39:9 (September 2008): 2611–2613.

22. Kull, I., A. Bergstrom, E. Melen, et al. "Early-life Supplementation of Vitamins A and D, in Water-soluble Form or in Peanut Oil, and Allergic Diseases during Childhood." *J Allergy Clin Immunol* 118:6 (December 2006): 1299– 1304.

23. Hypponen, E., U. Sovio, M. Wjst, et al. "Infant Vitamin D Supplementation and Allergic Conditions in Adulthood: Northern Finland Birth Cohort 1966." *Ann N Y Acad Sci* 1037 (December 2004): 84–95.

24. Hypponen, E., D.J. Berry, M. Wjst, C. Power. "Serum 25-Hydroxyvitamin D and IgE- A Significant but Nonlinear Relationship." *Allergy* 64:4 (April 2009): 613–620.

25. Camargo Jr., C.A., S. Clark, M.S. Kaplan, et al. "Regional Differences in EpiPen Prescriptions in the United States: The Potential Role of Vitamin D." *J Allergy Clin Immunol* 120:1 (July 2007): 131–136.

26. Brehm, J.M., and J.C. Celedón. "Serum Vitamin D Levels and Markers of Severity of Childhood Asthma in Costa Rica." *Am J Resp Crit Care Med* 179 (2009): 765–771.

27. Worm, M. "Novel Therapies for Atopic Eczema." *Curr Opin Investig Drugs* 3:11 (2002): 1596–1603.

28. Adorini, L., and G. Penna. "Control of Autoimmune Diseases by the Vitamin D Endocrine System." *Nat Clin Pract Rheumatol* 4:8 (August 2008): 404–412.

29. Kong, J., Z. Zhang, et al. "Novel Role of the Vitamin D Receptor in Maintaining the Integrity of the Intestinal Mucosal Barrier." *Am J Physiol Gastrointest Liver Physiol* 294:1 (January 2008): G208–G216.

30. Ekici, F., B. Ozyurt, H. Erdogan. "The Combination of Vitamin D3 and Dehydroascorbic Acid Administration Attenuates Brain Damage in Focal Ischemia." *Neurol Sci* 30:3 (June 2009): 207–212.

31. Grant, W.B. "An Estimate of Premature Cancer Mortality in the U.S. Because of Inadequate Doses of Solar Ultraviolet-B Radiation." *Cancer* 94:6 (2002): 1867–1875.

32. Aloia, J.F., and M. Li-Ng. "Epidemic Influenza and Vitamin D." *Epidemiol Infect* 135 (2007): 1095–1096.

33. Mann, G.V., et al. "Atherosclerosis in the Maasai." *Am J Epidemiol* 95 (1972): 26–37. Mann, G.V. (ed.). *Coronary Heart Disease: The Dietary Sense and Nonsense.* London: Veritas Society, 1993, p. 1.

34. Freed, D.L.J. "Adipose Tissue and Adipokines in Health and Disease. Book Review." *J Nutr Environ Med* 17:2 (2008): 136–137.

35. [No authors listed.] "Multiple Risk Factor Intervention Trial. Risk Factor Changes and Mortality Results. Multiple Risk Factor Intervention Trial Research Group." *JAMA* 248:12 (September 1982): 1465–1477.

36. Hu, F.B., M.J. Stampfer, J.E. Manson, et al. "Dietary Fat Intake and the Risk of Coronary Heart Disease in Women." *New Engl J Med* 337:21 (1997): 1491–1499.

37. Chavarro, J.E., J.W. Rich-Edwards, B.A. Rosner, W.C. Willett. "Dietary Fatty Acid Intakes and the Risk of Ovulatory Infertility." *Am J Clin Nutr* 85:1 (2007): 231–237.

38. Mozaffarian, D., M.B. Katan, A. Ascherio, et al. "Trans-fatty Acids and Cardiovascular Disease." *N Engl J Med* 354:15 (2006): 1601–1613.

39. Chajès, V.A., C.M. Thiébaut, M. Rotival, et al. "Serum Trans-Monosaturated Fatty Acids are Associated with an Increased Risk of Breast Cancer in the E3N-EPIC Study." *Am J Epidemiol* 167 (2008): 1312.

40. Chavarro, J., M. Stampfer, H. Campos, et al. "A Prospective Study of Blood Trans Fatty Acid Levels and Risk of Prostate Cancer." *Proc Am Assoc Cancer Res* 47:1 (2006): 943.

41. Morris, M.C., D.A. Evans, J.L. Bienias, et al. "Dietary Fats and the Risk of Incident Alzheimer Disease." *Arch Neurol* 60:2 (2003): 194–200.

42. Belury, M. "Dietary Conjugated Linoleic Acid in Health: Physiological Effects and Mechanisms of Action." *Annu Rev Nutr* 22 (2002): 505–531.

43. Colin, A., J. Reggers, V. Castronovo, et al. "Lipids, Depression and Suicide." *Encephale* 29:1 (2003): 49–58.

44. Goldstein, R. "FDA Chooses Drug Industry Health Over Public Health." February 23, 2005. CommonDreams.org. Available online at: www.commondreams.org/views05/0223-35.htm.

45. Yehuda, S., and R.L. Carasso. "Effects of Dietary Fats on Learning, Pain Threshold, Thermoregulation and Motor Activity in Rats: Interaction with the Length of Feeding Period." *Int J Neurosci* 32:3–4 (February 1987): 919–925. Yehuda, S., S. Rabinovitz, D.I. Mostofsky, et al. "Essential Fatty Acid Preparation Improves Biochemical and Cognitive Functions in Experimental Allergic Encephalomyelitis Rats." *Eur J Pharmacol* 328:1 (June 1997): 23–29.

46. Ibid.

47. Dominguez L.G., M. Barbagallo, G. Di Lorenzo, et al. "Bronchial Reactivity and Intracellular Magnesium: A Possible Mechanism for the Bronchodilating Effects of Magnesium in Asthma." *Clin Sci* 95 (1998): 137–142.

48. Rea, W.J., A.R. Johnson, R.E. Smiley, et al. "Magnesium Deficiency in Patients with Chemical Sensitivity." *Clin Ecol* 4:1 (1986): 17–20.

49. Myhill, S., N.E. Booth, J. McLaren-Howard. "Chronic Fatigue Syndrome and Mitochondrial Dysfunction." *Int J Clin Exp Med* 2 (2009): 1–16.

50. Rowe, A.H. "A Synergism of Antigen Challenge and Severe Magnesium Deficiency in Blood and Urinary Histamine Levels in Rats." *J Am Coll Nutr* 9 (1990): 616–622.

51. Britton, J., I. Pavord, K. Richards, et al. "Dietary Magnesium, Lung Function, Wheezing, and Airway Hyper-reactivity in a Random Adult Population Sample." *Lancet* 344 (1994): 357–362.

52. Rowe, B.H., and C.A. Camargo Jr. "The Role of Magnesium Sulfate in the Acute and Chronic Management of Asthma." *Curr Opin Pulm Med* 14:1 (2008): 70–76.

Chapter 7: Exercise and Lifestyle Changes

1. Jackson, A., J. Morrow, D. Hill, R. Dishman. *Physical Activity for Health and Fitness*. Champaign, IL: Human Kinetics, 2003.

2. Hu, F., J. Manson, M. Stampfer, et al. "Diet, Lifestyle, and the Risk of Type 2 Diabetes Mellitus in Women." *New Engl J Med* 345:11 (2001): 790–797.

3. American Cancer Society. www.cancer.org.

4. Elwood, J.M., et al. "Sun Exposure and Malignant Melanoma." *Br J Cancer* 51 (1985): 543–549.

Chapter 8: Desensitization and Other Options

1. Miller, Joseph B. *Food Allergy: Provocative Testing and Injection Therapy*. Springfield, IL: Charles C. Thomas, 1972.

2. Jewett, D.L., G. Fein, M.H. Greenberg. "A Double-blind Study of Symptom Provocation to Determine Food Sensitivity." *New Engl J Med* 23 (1990): 429–433.

3. Miller, J. "A Double-blind Study of Food Extract Injection Therapy." *Ann Allergy* 38 (1977): 185–191. Scadding, G.K., and J. Brostoff. "Low-dose Sublingual Therapy in Patients with Allergic Rhinitis Due to House Dust Mite." *Clin Allergy* 16 (1986): 483–491. King, W.P., R.G. Fadal, W.A. Ward, et al. "Provocation/Neutralisation: A Two-part Study. Part II. Subcutaneous Neutralization Therapy: A Multi-center Study." *Otolaryngol Head Neck Surg* 99 (1988): 272–277.

4. Di Stanislao, C., E. Mazzocchetti, G. Bologna, S. Chimenti. "EPD secondo McEwen: Studio clinico, istologico e immunoistochimico." *Boll Dermatol Allergol Prof* 2 (1994). Longo, G., F. Poli, G. Bertoli. "Efficacia clinica di un nuovo trattamento iposensibilizzante, EPD (Enzime Potentiated Desensitisation) nella terapia della pollinosi." *Riforma Med* 107 (1992): 171–176. Astarita, C., G. Scala, S. Sproviero, A. Franzese. "A Double-blind Placebo-controlled Trial of Enzyme Potentiated Desensitisation in the Treatment of Pollenosis." *J Invest Allergol Clin Immunol* 6:4 (1996): 248–255. Angelini, G., G. Curatoli, V. D'Argento, G.A. Vena. "Pollinosi: Una nuova metodica di immunoterapia." *Mediterr J Surg Med* (1993): 253–256. Cantani, A., M.A. Monteleone, V. Ragno, et al. "Enzyme Potentiated Desensitisation in Children with Asthma and Mite Allergy: A Double-blind Study." *J Invest Allergol Clin Immunol* 6:4 (1996): 270–276. Ippoliti, F., V. Ragno, A. Del Nero, et al. "Effect of Preseasonal Enzyme Potentiated Desensitisation (EPD) on Plasma IL-6 and IL-10 of Grass Pollen-sensitive Asthmatic Children." *Allergie Immunol* 29:5 (1997): 120, 123–125.

5. Radcliffe M.J., G.T. Lewith, R.G. Turner, et al. "Enzyme Potentiated Desensitisation in Treatment of Allergic Rhinitis: Double-blind Randomised Controlled Study." *Br Med J* 327 (August 2003): 251–254.

INDEX

ABOUT THE AUTHOR

Damien Downing, M.D., is president of the British Society for Ecological Medicine and editor of the *Journal of Nutritional and Environmental Medicine*. Since 1980, his work has established him as a leading figure in nutritional medicine in the U.K. He has undertaken pioneering work in the treatment of allergy, the linking of behavioral disorders with nutrition, and light therapy and the treatment of chronic fatigue, autism, and attention deficit/hyperactivity disorder. Dr. Downing maintains a private practice in the U.K. focusing on nutritional and alternative therapies.

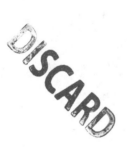